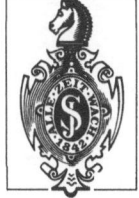

W. Braune   O. Fischer

Determination of the Moments of Inertia of the Human Body and Its Limbs

Translators:
P. Maquet   R. Furlong

With 12 Figures and 15 Tables

Springer-Verlag Berlin Heidelberg GmbH

Wilhelm Braune †   Otto Fischer †

Translators:

Dr. Paul Maquet
25, Thier Bosset, B-4070 Aywaille, Belgium

Ronald Furlong, M.B., B.S., F.R.C.S
149, Harley Street, GB-London W1N 2DE,
United Kingdom

The manuscript of this work was begun by both authors some days before the
death of Prof. Dr. W. Braune.

Title of the original German edition: Bestimmung der Trägheitsmomente des
menschlichen Körpers und seiner Glieder. Published by S. Hirzel, Leipzig, 1892.

ISBN 978-3-662-11238-0   ISBN 978-3-662-11236-6 (eBook)
DOI 10.1007/978-3-662-11236-6

Library of Congress Cataloging-in-Publication Data
Braune, Wilhelm, 1831–1892. Determination of the moments of inertia of the human
body and its limbs. Translation of: Bestimmung der Trägheitsmomente des menschlichen
Körpers und seiner Glieder. Leipzig: S. Hirzel, 1892. Includes Index. 1. Human mechanics. 2. Moments of inertia. I. Fischer, O. (Otto), 1861–1916. II. Title. [DNLM:
1. Biophysics. 2. Movements. 3. Reflex-physiology. QT 34 B825b] QP303.B7313   1988
612'.76 88-2028

© Springer-Verlag Berlin Heidelberg 1988
Originally published by Springer-Verlag Berlin Heidelberg New York in 1988

2124/3140-543210

Preface

This is another classic contribution by Braune and Fischer to the field of biomechanics.

The pendulum method was employed to ascertain accurately the moments and radii of inertia of the human body and its different parts about all axes – transverse, oblique or longitudinal. This elegant method is described in detail, together with the results. Relations were found between the centres of inertia on one hand and the lengths and diameters of the body segments on the other. These data were originally prepared for the authors' later work, *The Human Gait,* to determine the forces exerted on and by the parts of the body during walking.

Such work is the basis for solving the mechanical problems related to any movement of the human body: thus, the original results presented here continue to be of immense value to current research and practice.

Aywaille, May 1988   P. Maquet

Contents

Introduction

𝔄 ny movement of a rigid body can be resolved into two components: displacement and rotation. A movement is called displacement when all the points of the body describe parallel straight lines. Rotation occurs when the points of a straight line of the body designated as the axis of rotation do not change position and all the other points describe circles the centres of which are on the axis of rotation and the planes of which are at right angles to this axis.

Any change in location of a rigid body consists of a displacement of any one of its points and a simultaneous rotation about a straight line through this point. This point of the body can be chosen at will. In general, for any other point, the magnitude of the displacement, the direction of the axis through this point and the magnitude of the rotation are different. Particularly the point can be chosen such that the axis of rotation coincides with the direction of the displacement. In such an instance the combination of the two components of the movement is called helical movement and the axis of rotation the helical axis. On the other hand, the centre of gravity of the body can also be chosen. Then the change in location combines a displacement of the centre of gravity with a rotation about a straight line through this centre of gravity.

Determination of the displacement and rotation which correspond to a finite change in location of the body, however, does not give any insight into the actual progress of the movement between the two extreme locations. To know this progress, the change in location must be imagined as being resolved into a sufficient number of very small changes in location of the body, more precisely into an infinite number of infinitely small shifts.

For the particular goal of the present study it is important to know which point of the body has to be selected to carry out the small shifts.

If only a clear representation of the process of the movement in a kinematic sense is required, without considering its causes, it is conve-

1

nient to choose the point such that the small displacement occurs in the direction of the axis of rotation. Then the movement of the body is resolved into a sequence of very small helical movements. The helical axes corresponding to the successive helical movements (instant axes) generally have different positions in the body but they are very close to each other and form a ruled surface, that is a surface constituted by a series of straight lines. Each of the successive helical axes of the moving body during the small helical movement about it momentarily coincides with a fixed straight line in space. All these fixed straight lines in space also form a ruled surface different from the first. The latter remains fixed in space during the movement of the body. The former changes its position in space since it is linked to the moving body. At each instant a straight line of the moving ruled surface coincides with one of the fixed one. That is the straight line which is used as the helical axis at this instant. Consequently, during the movement of the body, one ruled surface rolls over the other which is fixed in space, and simultaneously slides over the straight lines which coincide. Using the two ruled surfaces illustrates very well the geometrical process of the movement.

To investigate how the movement of the body originates through the forces applied to it (dynamics), it is convenient to choose the centre of gravity of the body for each shift and to consider the movement as a consequence of small displacements of the centre of gravity combined with simultaneous rotation about a straight line through this centre of gravity. Generally then both the direction of the displacement and the direction of the axis of rotation change continuously and are different from each other at each instant. If infinitely small shifts are considered, the centre of gravity describes a curve in space and the axes of rotation form a cone fixed to the body. The apex of this cone coincides with the centre of gravity. This resolution of the movement of a rigid body is mechanically important. According to the differential movement equations, when a rigid body is moved by external forces, the movement of its centre of gravity proceeds as if the total mass of the body were concentrated at the centre of gravity and all the external forces applied at the body were displaced parallel to themselves towards the centre of gravity. If the lines of action of all the forces pass through the centre of gravity, the movement of the body actually consists of a movement of the centre of gravity without simultaneous rotation about any axis through the centre of gravity. In such an instance, all the forces are combined into a resultant applied at the centre of gravity. The problem is restricted to the determination of the movement of a point under the effect of a force applied at this point.

If, as is usual, the lines of action of the forces are at a distance from the centre of gravity, the forces tend to rotate the body about an axis through the centre of gravity.

Any body is subjected to inertia, which tends to maintain its state of rest or movement. Therefore, it offers some resistance to all forces which tend to change its state of movement. This resistance is different when a force tends to displace the body from when a force tends to rotate it.

The state of movement of a body is expressed by its velocity, the direction and magnitude of which the body tends to maintain. Rest is a particular state of the state of movement which is characterized by a zero velocity. Apart from a change in direction, a modification in the magnitude of the state of movement of a body consists of either an increase or a decrease of its velocity. The increase or decrease in velocity which the body would experience if the cause of the change in its state acted evenly on the body during 1 s is called acceleration. The acceleration is positive when velocity is increased and negative when velocity is decreased.

When the body is displaced, velocity and acceleration (or displacement velocity and displacement acceleration) are linear. When there is rotation about an axis, velocity and acceleration are angular (or rotatory velocity and rotatory acceleration).

Linear velocity and acceleration are measured by vectors in relation to a point of the body. Angular velocity and acceleration are measured by arcs described by any point of the body at distance 1 from the axis of rotation.

It is a fundamental problem of dynamics to analyse: on one hand, the changes in the state of movement which forces applied to the body tend to impart to the body, as a result of their magnitudes, directions and points of application; on the other hand, the resistance with which the body opposes the action of these forces as a result of its inertia.

The analysis will be restricted to the two types of movement, displacement and rotation, from which all the other movements result and to the behaviour of the centre of gravity of a body towards external forces. The problem thus is resolved into four questions which can be grouped in pairs depending on whether they relate to displacement or to rotation.

1. Displacement:
a) What linear acceleration does a force applied at its centre of gravity tend to impart to a rigid body?

b) With what resistance does the body oppose this acceleration tendency as a result of its inertia?

2. Rotation:

a) What angular acceleration does a force, applied somewhere, tend to impart to a body susceptible to rotation about a fixed axis?

b) With what resistance does the body oppose this acceleration tendency as a result of its inertia[1]?

The rules are as follows:

1. Displacement:

a) The greater the force the greater the tendency to evoke a linear acceleration. The acceleration is proportional to the magnitude of the force. *Thus the magnitude of the force is a direct measure of the tendency of this force to impart a linear acceleration to the body.* If several forces are applied at the centre of gravity, their resultant is a measure of the resultant tendency to acceleration.

b) The greater the mass of the body the greater the resistance offered by the body. This resistance is proportional to the magnitude of the mass. *Thus the magnitude of the mass of a body is a direct measure of the resistance offered by this body to the tendency of the forces to impart to it a linear acceleration.*

Consequently, the actual linear acceleration must be in direct proportion to the magnitude of the forces exerted and in inverse proportion to the magnitude of the mass of the body. If the linear acceleration is designated as b, the resultant force as K and the mass of the body as M, the following relationship exists between these magnitudes for a proper choice of the units:

$$b = \frac{K}{M}.$$

2. Rotation:

a) In rotation, generally only part of the force takes effect. In order to determine this part, the force must be resolved into two components, one in the direction of the axis of rotation and the other at right angles to the first. Only the latter tends to rotate the body about the fixed axis. The magnitude of this tendency depends on the magnitude of the

---

[1] Only these four simple instances will be considered here, without mentioning normal acceleration and resistance of the body against changes in direction (centrifugal force), to avoid expanding these introductory remarks further than necessary for the present aim which consists of elucidating the concept of the moment of inertia and its importance for dynamics.

acting component, on the distance between the point of application of this component and the axis of rotation, i.e. the lever of the force, and on the angle formed by this force and the direction of the lever. The tendency of the force to rotate is the greater the greater the component of the force at right angles to the axis of rotation, the longer its lever and the greater the acute angle formed by the direction of the acting component and the lever. The tendency to rotate is proportional to the magnitude of the component of the force, the length of the lever and the sine of the angle formed by the lever and the component of the force. If the magnitude of the acting component of the force is designated as K, the lever as h and the angle formed by the lever and the component of the force as α, the tendency of the force to rotate is proportional to $K h \sin \alpha$. In mechanics this expression is called moment of rotation of the force or torque. *The torque is a measure of the tendency of the force to impart to the body an angular acceleration about a given axis of rotation.*

The magnitude of the torque can be arrived at in two different ways.

It can be asked how great a force acting at right angles to a lever 1 is necessary to evoke the same tendency to rotate as the given force does with its actual lever. The magnitude of this force is generally different from that of the acting component. It can be expressed as $K h \sin \alpha$. Then the torque is:

$$(K h \sin \alpha) \cdot 1 \cdot \sin 90° = K h \sin \alpha.$$

The torque is the same as that of the given force. This representation of the torque is usually considered a definition of the torque although this is not correct since force and torque have different dimensions.

Another way of representing the magnitude of the torque is more geometrical. It consists of indicating the lever at right angles to the acting component of the force which is necessary to evoke the same tendency to rotate as this component does when inclined to the actual lever. This segment is called the lever arm of the force. Its length is $h \sin \alpha$. Then the force K which acts at right angles to the lever arm $h \sin \alpha$ produces the torque:

$$K \cdot (h \sin \alpha) \cdot \sin 90° = K h \sin \alpha.$$

This is the same as that of the force acting with its actual lever and direction. If the lever arm is called i, the magnitude of the torque due to the component of the force K is $K i$. If several forces are applied to the body, the several torques combine into one resultant tendency to rotate.

b) The tendency of a force to rotate depends not only on the magnitude of this force but also on the position of the axis of rotation in the body. Similarly, the resistance offered by the mass of the body to the tendency of the forces to impart an angular acceleration depends on the magnitude of the mass of the body and on the position of the axis of rotation in the body. The greater the mass of a body the greater its resistance. The resistance thus is proportional to the magnitude of the mass. To recognize the influence of the position of the axis of rotation on the resistance, the mass must be conceived as being resolved into a great number of very small masses. The resistance then is also resolved into as many small resistances. All the small individual masses do not participate in the overall resistance equally even if their magnitudes are equal. All the small masses rotate with the same angular velocity and the rotating force imparts to them the same angular acceleration. However, the linear velocities and accelerations which they display in the direction of the tangents to their curved trajectories at a given instant are very different. The further a small mass lies from the axis of rotation, the longer its trajectory during rotation and consequently the greater its linear velocity at this instant. When the angular velocity changes, the small masses very distant from the axis of rotation display a greater change in their linear velocity than do those near the axis and, consequently, they offer more resistance to rotation. The resistance of a small mass is not simply proportional to its distance from the axis of rotation but is proportional to the square of this distance.

This can be illustrated as follows:

Two isolated small masses are assumed to be the one at a distance 1 and the other at a distance r from the axis of rotation. The same torque d acts on both. On the first small mass the force acts at right angles to the lever arm 1. The magnitude of this force thus is d. On the second small mass the force acts at right angles to the lever arm r. This force thus must be equal to $\dfrac{d}{r}$ since it exerts the same torque d. In both instances the force is applied to the mass itself. Therefore, the linear acceleration is $\dfrac{d}{m}$ for the first mass and $\dfrac{d}{rm}$ for the second mass. The linear acceleration of the small mass at a distance r from the axis thus is only the $\dfrac{1}{r}$ part of the linear acceleration of the small mass at a distance 1 from the axis. If the two linear accelerations were equal, then the angular accelerations would be different. The mass at a distance r from the axis would display an angular acceleration r times smaller than the mass at a distance 1 since, for the same angle, the arcs on the circle with radius r are r times longer than those on the circle with radius 1. However, the linear acceleration of the mass at a distance r from the axis is r times smaller than that of the other mass. Therefore, its angular acceleration is rr or r^2 smaller than that of the mass at a distance 1 from the axis. Since the torques are equal, the discrepancy in angular acceleration can result only from the fact that the mass at a distance r from the axis opposes the tendency of the force to rotate with an r^2 greater resistance. This resistance actually is proportional to the square of the distance of the mass from the axis of rotation. The resistance is also proportional to the magnitude of the mass m. Consequently, the expression mr^2 is a measure of the resistance offered by a small mass at a distance r from the axis of rotation to the tendency of a force to rotate the body. Adding the expressions mr^2 for all the small masses of the body gives the total resistance T of the whole body for the axis under consideration:

$$T = \sum mr^2$$

or, if the body is continuous:

$$T = \int r^2\, dm \quad \text{or} \quad \iiint r^2 \mu\, dx\, dy\, dz$$

μ is the density at point x, y, z. This magnitude has been termed by Euler: "moment of inertia of the body about the axis of rotation". *"The moment of inertia of a body about a given axis of rotation is a measure of the resistance which the body offers to the tendency of forces to rotate it about this axis".*

The magnitude of the moment of inertia can be conceived in two ways.

One consists of determining what mass must be put at a distance 1 from the axis of rotation in order to obtain the same resistance against rotation as that displayed by all the masses of the body at their actual distances. Putting the mass at a distance 1 from the axis of rotation is equivalent to placing this mass on the surface of a cylinder the axis of which is the axis of rotation and the radius is 1. The magnitude of this mass generally is different from that of the mass of the body and is expressed directly by $\sum mr^2$. Its moment of inertia is:

$$(\sum mr^2) \cdot 1^2 = \sum mr^2.$$

It is the same as that of the body.

As for the torque, it is usual directly to give this expression of the moment of inertia as its definition. However, this is not correct since the mass and the moment of inertia have different dimensions.

7

A more geometrical way of expressing the magnitude of the moment of inertia consists of indicating the distance from the axis at which the actual mass of the body must be concentrated in order to offer the same resistance against rotation as do all the small masses at their actual distances from the axis. This distance is called radius of inertia about the axis of rotation. Its magnitude is:

$$\sqrt{\frac{\sum m r^2}{\sum m}}$$

The overall mass $\sum m$ when put at this distance has a moment of inertia:

$$\sum m \cdot \left(\sqrt{\frac{\sum m r^2}{\sum m}} \right) = \sum m r^2.$$

This is the same as that obtained with the different small masses taken together. If the radius of inertia is called $\varkappa$ and the total mass $\sum m$ is called M, the moment of inertia is:

$$T = M \varkappa^2.$$

This expression of the magnitude of the moment of inertia by a vector presents the drawback that the vector is not proportional to the moment of inertia itself but is proportional to its square root. However, it is clearer than the representation of the torque by the lever arm. Therefore, it will be used mostly and the moment of inertia will be considered as determined when the radius of inertia is known.

Thus it appears that the actual angular acceleration of a body rotating about a fixed axis must be in direct proportion to the magnitude of the torque of the acting force and in inverse proportion to the magnitude of the moment of inertia of the body, both related to the axis of rotation. If the angular acceleration is designated as w, the resultant torque as R and the moment of inertia as T, for a proper choice of the units, these three magnitudes relate to each other as follows:

$$w = \frac{R}{T}.$$

Torque and moment of inertia play the same role in rotation as force and mass do in displacement.

All movements of a body can be conceived as displacements and rotations. For this conception in the sense of dynamics, the centre of gravity of the body is of decisive importance. Therefore, the movement of a body can be determined if one knows:

1. the magnitude of the motive forces, their position in relation to the centre of gravity of the body and their torque about any axis in space;
2. the mass of the body to be moved, the position of its centre of gravity and its moments of inertia about all axes in space.

Therefore, the behaviour of the body to be moved, towards the acting forces, is as important and necessary to analyse as the magnitudes of the forces and their torques. To this end one must determine

1. the mass of the body,
2. the position of its centre of gravity and
3. its moments of inertia about all axes in space.

These three points completely characterize a body from a mechanical point of view. Two bodies for which these three points are the same are mechanically equivalent even if they are very different in shape and constitution.

Analysis of the dynamics of the human body requires determination of these three points for the object of the movement, i.e. the different segments of the body. Masses and centres of gravity of the parts of the human body have been determined. The moments of inertia, however, have not yet been analysed, as far as we know.

Therefore, we assigned ourselves the goal of determining the moments of inertia about all possible axes in space, at least for the largest segments of the human body.

Experimental Determination of the Moments of Inertia of the Parts of the Body About Axes Through the Centre of Gravity and at Right Angles to the Longitudinal Axis, and About the Longitudinal Axis Itself

*T*he magnitude of a moment of inertia cannot generally be calculated. It can, however, be calculated in homogeneous bodies of geometrically defined form. Then the moment of inertia is determined by integral calculus. It can also be calculated for some bodies of uneven density when the latter changes in such a way that the body can be conceived as a steady sequence of homogeneous concentric spherical shells. Then, as shown by Schlömilch, the moments of inertia of bodies of revolution can be reduced to those of spheres or spherical shells of finite thickness.

But in bodies like the human body, the magnitudes of the moments of inertia can be deduced only empirically.

Usually the moment of inertia is determined by measuring oscillations of the body suspended by an elastic wire or by two threads. If the moment of inertia of a magnet is to be found, the magnet is suspended in such a way that it can oscillate about a vertical axis and the oscillating period τ_1 is observed. Then the moment of inertia is increased by a known magnitude T', for instance by adding either two equal masses at the same distance from the axis of rotation or a ring of known dimensions and mass placed concentrically about the axis of rotation. The magnet thus loaded is swung again and the oscillating period τ_2 is measured. The moment of inertia can be deduced from the three magnitudes τ_1, τ_2 and T' without taking into account the dimensions of the magnet. The rules valid for a physical pendulum with equal torques are applied. Thus:

$$\frac{\tau_1^2}{\tau_2^2} = \frac{T}{T + T'}$$

$$T = T' \frac{\tau_1^2}{\tau_2^2 - \tau_1^2}.$$

Despite its simplicity and the little calculation required, this method is not suitable for analysing the different parts of the human body.

After some preliminaries we devised the following method. As for determining the centres of gravity, we froze the body hard and oscillated its different segments as pendulums about horizontal axes through the centres of the joints. The duration of an oscillation was measured as well as the weight and the distance between the centre of gravity and the axis. From these three magnitudes the moment of inertia about this axis could be deduced. It was not necessary to observe the duration of an oscillation for the moment of inertia increased by a known quantity.

The moment of inertia of the body about the fixed axis is designated as T, the distance between the centre of gravity and the axis as e and the mass of the oscillating body as M. According to the rules for the pendulum, the period of an oscillation is:

$$\tau = \pi \sqrt{\frac{T}{M\,g\,e}}$$

where g is the terrestrial acceleration.

Thus:

$$T = \frac{\tau^2\,M\,g\,e}{\pi^2}.$$

The moments of inertia of a body about all the axes in space are known when the moments of inertia about all the axes through the centre of gravity are known.

If T_0 is the moment of inertia about an axis through the centre of gravity of the body and T the moment of inertia about an axis parallel to and at a distance e from the former (Fig. 1), the following equation pertains:

$$T = T_0 + M\,e^2.$$

This can be demonstrated. $A_0\,B_0$ is an axis through the centre of gravity S_0 of the body, AB an axis parallel to and at a distance e from $A_0\,B_0$; P is a point the mass of which is m; $PQ_0 = r$ is the distance of this point from the axis $A_0\,B_0$ and $PQ = \varrho$ its distance from the axis AB; $RQ_0 = PN = p$ is the projection of the segment PQ_0 on the line $Q_0\,Q = \varrho$. The following equation pertains:

$$\varrho^2 = r^2 + e^2 - 2\,e\,p.$$

12

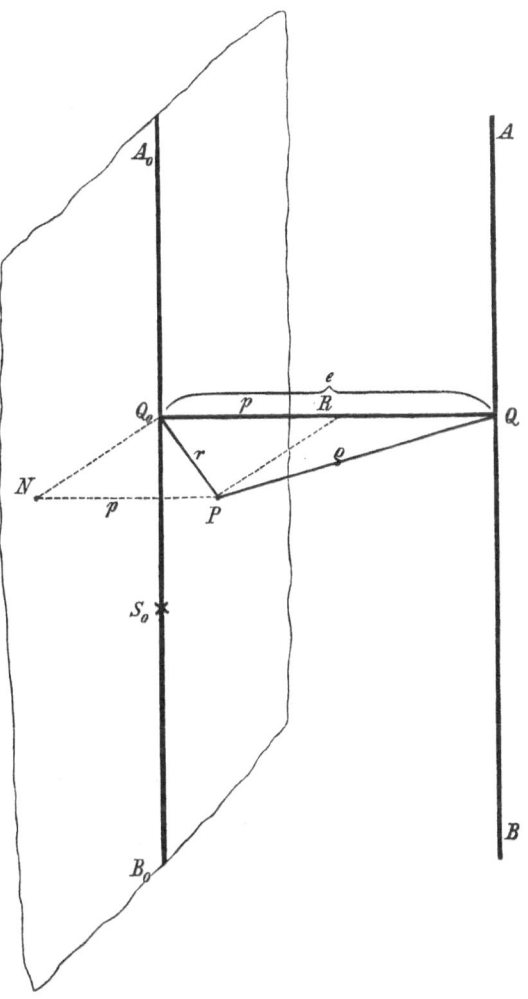

Fig. 1. Determination of the moment of inertia of a body about an axis AB parallel to another axis $A_0 B_0$ through the centre of gravity S_0

The moment of inertia of the punctual mass P is $m r^2$ about the axis $A_0 B_0$ and $m \varrho^2$ about the axis AB. If the moments of inertia of all the punctual masses of the body about the two axes are established, the total moment of inertia is in any case the summation of the moments of inertia of the different punctual masses. If T_0 designates the moment of inertia of the whole body about the axis $A_0 B_0$ through the centre of gravity and T the moment of inertia about the axis AB, the following equations pertain:

13

$$T_0 = \sum m r^2$$

and

$$T = \sum m \varrho^2$$

or

$$T = \sum m (r^2 + e^2 - 2 e p)$$

where e is a constant. Therefore, the value of T can also be written as:

$$T = \sum m r^2 + e^2 \cdot \sum m - 2 e \sum m p.$$

In this equation $\sum m r^2$ is the moment of inertia T_0 about the axis $A_0 B_0$, $\sum m$ is the mass M of the whole body and $\sum m p$ is the summation of the products of the mass of each individual point and its distance from a fixed plane through $A_0 B_0$. Since this plane is through the centre of gravity, this sum is 0. It is a property of the centre of gravity that the masses on both sides of a plane through this centre of gravity are equal as long as the summation of the products of the mass of each point and its distance from the plane is equal on both sides. Their algebraic sum thus is 0. Therefore:

$$T = T_0 + M e^2.$$

If $\varkappa_0$ is the radius of inertia about the axis through the centre of gravity, the following equation pertains:

$$T_0 = M \varkappa_0^2$$

and, consequently:

$$T = M (\varkappa_0^2 + e^2).$$

Introducing this value in the above equation to determine T gives an equation for determining the radius of inertia $\varkappa_0$ about an axis through the centre of gravity and parallel to the axis of oscillation.

$$M (\varkappa_0^2 + e^2) = \frac{\tau^2 M g e}{\pi^2}$$

$$\varkappa_0 = \frac{1}{\pi} \sqrt{(g \tau^2 - \pi^2 e) e}$$

It is necessary experimentally to find the duration of an oscillation τ and the distance e between the axis of oscillation and the centre of gravity to enable the radius of inertia $\varkappa_0$ about an axis through the centre of gravity and parallel to the axis of oscillation to be calculated.

14

Knowing the magnitude of the mass M is not necessary to find the radius of inertia although it is necessary to find the moment of inertia itself.

Direct measurement of e is always inaccurate because the centre of gravity is usually inside the body segment. This measurement can be disposed of if the body is suspended successively from two parallel axes in a plane comprising the centre of gravity.

τ_1 is the period of oscillation about an axis and e_1 the distance between this axis and the centre of gravity. τ_2 and e_2 are their counterparts for the oscillation about the other axis.

$$\tau_1 = \pi \sqrt{\frac{\varkappa_0^2 + e_1^2}{g\,e_1}}$$

$$\tau_2 = \pi \sqrt{\frac{\varkappa_0^2 + e_2^2}{g\,e_2}}$$

$$e_1 + e_2 = l$$

l is the distance between the two axes.

From these three equations it appears that:

$$e_1 = \frac{(\pi^2\,l - g\,\tau_2^2)\,l}{2\,\pi^2\,l - g\,(\tau_1^2 + \tau_2^2)}$$

$$e_2 = \frac{(\pi^2\,l - g\,\tau_1^2)\,l}{2\,\pi^2\,l - g\,(\tau_2^2 + \tau_1^2)}$$

Consequently:

$$\varkappa_0 = \frac{1}{\pi}\sqrt{(g\,\tau_1^2 - \pi^2\,e_1)\,e_1}$$

and

$$\varkappa_0 = \frac{1}{\pi}\sqrt{(g\,\tau_2^2 - \pi^2\,e_2)\,e_2}.$$

This provides a check for the calculation.

The period of the pendulum can be measured fairly accurately only by observing a great number of oscillations of small amplitude. This enables the radius of inertia to be determined with as much accuracy

15

as that attained by measuring the distance l between the two axes. At the same time the position of the centre of gravity which has been determined experimentally can be checked.

In the first experiments we generally did not suspend the body segments from two axes and were satisfied with the direct measurement of the position of the centre of gravity.

First Series of Experiments

A normally built and strong man committed suicide. The cadaver was frozen stiff. The body segments were separated at joint levels and weighed. The distances between their centre of gravity and the adjacent joints were measured. The periods of the oscillations about axes through the centres of the joints were determined. The directions of the axes are described below and Table 1 gives the results of all direct measurements.

The axes through the centres of the joints are numbered starting from 1 for each body segment. For example, they are numbered from 1 to 7 for the thigh and the upper arm. Their directions are as follows. The roman number indicates the body segment and the index the number of the axis.

I_1 Line connecting the centres of the two hip joints.

$II_1 - II_4$ Axes through the centre of the hip joint in a plane at right angles to the longitudinal axis of the thigh. Their directions appear in the schematic horizontal cross section of the right thigh (Fig. 2). The four axes are symmetrical for the left hip.

$III_1 - III_4$ Same axes as $II_1 - II_4$.

III_5 Axis of the knee.

III_6 Axis almost parallel to the longitudinal axis of the thigh at a distance of 10.0 cm from the centre of gravity of the thigh on the right side, of 8.5 cm on the left side. These data, however, are not totally reliable since suspension of the body segment somewhat modified the distance from the centre of gravity.

III_7 Axis almost parallel to the longitudinal axis of the thigh. Distance of the centre of gravity of the thigh from the axis: about 9.5 cm on the right side, about 10.0 cm on the left side.

IV_1 Axis of the knee.

V_1 Axis of the knee.

V_2 Axis of the ankle.

VI_1 Axis of the ankle.

16

Table 1. Data necessary to calculate the moments of inertia (first series of experiments)

Body segments		Weight (g)	Length (cm)	Distance of the centre of gravity		Period τ of a pendulum oscillation of small amplitude measured on 100 oscillations (s)						
				from above e_1	from below e_2	1	2	3	4	5	6	7
Trunk + head	{ r l	28 450	78.0	45.0	33.0	0.658	–	–	–	–	–	–
Leg	{ r	10 160	87.0	35.0	52.0	0.714	0.705	0.690	0.680	–	–	–
	l	10 680	87.0	35.0	52.0	0.708	0.714	0.716	0.690	–	–	–
Thigh	{ r	6 450	40.0	17.5	22.5	0.488	0.484	0.490	0.488	0.522	0.352	0.366
	l	6 990	40.0	16.5	23.5	0.488	0.496	0.488	0.500	0.534	0.346	0.364
Lower leg + foot	{ r	3 680	47.0	25.0	22.0	0.586	–	–	–	–	–	–
	l	3 670	47.0	25.0	22.0	0.584	–	–	–	–	–	–
Lower leg	{ r	2 680	39.0	16.5	22.5	0.474	0.518	–	–	–	–	–
	l	2 660	39.0	16.0	23.0	0.474	0.518	–	–	–	–	–
Foot	{ r	990	20.0	6.0	14.0	0.346	–	–	–	–	–	–
	l	1 000	20.0	6.0	14.0	0.354	–	–	–	–	–	–
Arm	{ r	3 160	65.0	26.0	39.0	0.616	0.620	0.616	0.606	–	–	–
	l	3 290	64.0	26.5	37.5	0.622	0.622	0.622	0.614	–	–	–
Upper arm	{ r	1 710	28.5	13.0	15.5	0.424	0.426	0.424	0.416	0.436	0.246	0.280
	l	1 850	29.5	13.5	16.0	0.430	0.410	0.426	0.426	0.448	0.260	0.268
Forearm + hand	{ r	1 440	37.0	17.0	20.0	0.474	–	–	–	–	–	–
	l	1 420	36.0	16.5	19.5	0.476	–	–	–	–	–	–
Whole body		58 500	165.0									

17

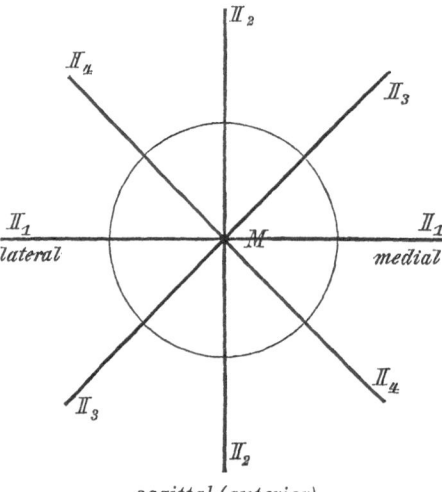

II_2

II_4

II_3

II_1
lateral

M

II_1
medial

II_3

II_4

II_2

sagittal (anterior)

Fig. 2. Horizontal cross section through the centre of the hip. M: centre of the hip. (As seen from above)

$VII_1 - VII_4$ Axes through the shoulder joint in a plane at right angles to the longitudinal axis of the upper arm. They correspond precisely to the axes $II_1 - II_4$ through the hip joint.

$VIII_1 - VIII_4$ Same axes as $VII_1 - VII_4$.

VIII_6 Axis almost parallel to the longitudinal axis of the upper arm. Its distance from the centre of gravity of the upper arm was about 6.0 cm on the right side and 5.5 cm on the left side. These data are as unreliable as those concerning the axes III_6 and III_7.

VIII_7 Axis approximately parallel to the longitudinal axis of the upper arm. Distance of this axis from the centre of gravity of the upper arm: on the right side about 5.5 cm, on the left side about 4.5 cm.

IX_1 Axis of the elbow.

In all instances in which the periods of oscillations about two parallel axes in the plane comprising the centre of gravity have been determined, the equations of p. 15 must be used to calculate the distances e_1 and e_2 between the centre of gravity and the centres of the adjacent joints. This enables data obtained by direct measurement to be checked.

This concerns the thigh, upper arm and lower leg. For the thigh and upper arm the axes 1 and 5, for the lower leg the axes 1 and 2 are

18

approximately parallel. The centre of gravity lies on the line connecting the centres of the joints at the extremities of the body segment[2], which is in the plane determined by the two parallel axes.

According to Table 1, for the right thigh:

$\tau_1 = 0.488$

$\tau_2 = 0.522$

$l = 40.0$.

Counting terrestrial acceleration as 980.8[3] gives a value of 17.7 cm for e_1 whereas direct measurement gave 17.5 cm.

For the left thigh:

$\tau_1 = 0.488$

$\tau_2 = 0.534$

$l = 40.0$.

Calculation gives $e_1 = 16.7$ cm whereas the directly measured value was 16.5 cm.

For the right upper arm:

$\tau_1 = 0.424$

$\tau_2 = 0.436$

$l = 28.5$.

Calculation gives $e_1 = 13.5$ cm whereas direct measurement had given 13.0 cm.

For the left upper arm:

$\tau_1 = 0.430$

$\tau_2 = 0.448$

$l = 29.5$.

Calculation gives $e_1 = 13.6$ cm whereas direct measurement had given $e = 13.5$ cm.

---

[2] Braune W, Fischer O (1984) On the centre of gravity of the human body. Springer, Berlin Heidelberg New York Tokyo.

[3] This value is valid only for the latitude of Paris. Its difference from that valid in Leipzig is not sufficient to impair the precision attainable in these first experiments. In later experiments the precise value valid in Leipzig was used (see p. 38).

For the right and left lower legs:

$$\tau_1 = 0.474$$
$$\tau_2 = 0.518$$
$$l = 39.0.$$

Calculation gives $e_1 = 16.6$ cm whereas direct measurement had given 16.5 cm for the right lower leg and 16.0 cm for the left.

Calculation of the distances from the centre of gravity to the centres of the joints in these six instances shows the best possible correspondence with direct measurements if the degree of accuracy of the latter is considered. Observation of the periods of oscillation about the two parallel axes in a plane in which the centre of gravity lies thus provides a new and more precise method of determining the position of the centre of gravity than the one which we used previously. Direct measurement of the distance between the two axes can be carried out more accurately than measurement of the distance between the centre of gravity located inside the body segment and one of the axes.

Using the equations on page 15 to calculate $\varkappa_0$ and the data of Table 1 (page 17) gives the radii and moments of inertia about the axes through the centre of gravity of a body segment (Table 2, p. 22).

Calculation has been carried out only for the radii of inertia about the coronal axis at right angles to the longitudinal axis and through the centre of gravity of the leg, thigh, arm and upper arm. The radii of inertia about the axes numbered 2, 3 and 4 in Table 1 have not been calculated. The periods of oscillation τ in relation to the four axes numbered 1–4 in the body segments and systems of body segments mentioned above show that the radii of inertia about these four axes are approximately the same. The periods of oscillation are little different and the differences do not have the same sign for the right and the left extremities. This cannot be due to a regular modification of the moment of inertia but must rather be attributed to errors. These errors can originate in the separation of the body segments or in the introduction of the axes. It can thus be stated that:

In the extremities and in their parts the moments of inertia about four axes and, as demonstrated later (pp. 56, 57), about all axes through the centre of gravity and at right angles to the longitudinal axis of the body segment are equal.

This is not true for the moment of inertia about the longitudinal axis of the body segment. This moment is smaller than those about the other axes. This results from the fact that the mass of the body segment is much closer to the longitudinal axis than to any other axis.

Determination of the radius of inertia about the longitudinal axis was less accurate in the first series of experiments because of the way the axes were placed. On one hand, as mentioned above, measurement of the distances between the centre of gravity and the axes was unreliable. On the other hand, for the axis in the vicinity of the centre of gravity a small error in measuring the distance from the centre of gravity exerts much greater effect on the accuracy of the result than for axes further away from the centre of gravity. Therefore, in every case two measurements were carried out about different axes and their average was taken. A significant source of error resulted from the fact that during the oscillation it was not possible to maintain parallel to the longitudinal axis the axes fixed in the soft parts which began to thaw somewhat. Although no great value can be attributed to these determinations of the moment of inertia about the longitudinal axis of the body segments, their magnitudes are given in Table 2 since they at least provide a provisional overall view for guidance.

The data in columns 3 and 6 of Table 2 enable the ratio of the radius of inertia about axes perpendicular to the longitudinal axis of the body segment to the length of the latter $\frac{\varkappa_0}{l}$ to be calculated (Table 3). This ratio is about the same for all body segments. Its average is 0.28 whether the trunk + head system is taken into account or not.

$\varkappa_0$ was calculated for the whole extremities and for their segments. Deducing the moment of inertia of a whole extremity from those of its segments provides a check of the measurements.

Two body segments are linked by a joint, as for instance (Fig. 3) the thigh and the lower leg + foot system (lower leg and foot being considered as one rigid mass). m_1 and m_2 designate the masses, $\varkappa_1$ and $\varkappa_2$ the radii of inertia about axes through the centres of gravity S_1 and S_2 of the body segments and parallel to the axis of the joint (axis of the knee), s_1 and s_2 the distances between the axis of the joint K and the centres of gravity S_1 and S_2. The distance d between the two centres of gravity was found using the following equation:

$$d^2 = s_1^2 + s_2^2 - 2\,s_1\,s_2 \cos\omega$$

in which ω is the angle formed by the lines connecting the centre of the joint K and the centres of gravity S_1 and S_2, i.e. the angle of flexion. The total centre of gravity S_0 lies on the line connecting S_1 and S_2 and divides this line in inverse proportion to the two masses. S_0 therefore

is at a distance $\dfrac{m_2}{m_1 + m_2}\,d$ from S_1 and at a distance $\dfrac{m_1}{m_1 + m_2}\,d$ from S_2.

Table 2. Radii and moments of inertia about axes through the centre of gravity of a body segment (first series of experiments)

Body segments		Mass (g)	Length l (cm)	Distance of the centre of gravity		Radius of inertia $\varkappa$ and moment of inertia $T = m\varkappa^2$ about axes through the centre of gravity			
				from above	from below	Axis at right angles to the long axis of the body segment		Long axis of the body segment	
				e_1 (cm)	e_2 (cm)	$\varkappa_0$ (cm)	$T = m\varkappa_0^2$ (cm²·g)	$\varkappa_0$ (cm)	$T = m\varkappa_0^2$ (cm²·g)
Trunk + head		28 450	78.0	45.0	33.0	18.2	9 417 000	–	–
Upper arm	r	1 710	28.5	13.5	15.0	7.7	101 000	1.8 (?)	–
	l	1 850	29.4	13.6	15.9	8.1	121 000	3.1	18 000
Forearm + hand	r	1 440	37.0	17.0	20.0	9.5	130 000	–	–
	l	1 420	36.0	16.5	19.5	10.0	142 000	–	–
Thigh	r	6 450	40.0	17.7	22.3	10.3	684 000	5.4	19 000
	l	6 990	40.0	16.7	23.3	10.8	818 000	5.5	21 000
Lower leg + foot	r	3 680	47.0	25.0	22.0	15.1	839 000	–	–
	l	3 670	47.0	25.0	22.0	14.9	814 000	–	–
Lower leg	r	2 680	39.0	16.5	22.5	9.8	257 000	–	–
	l	2 660	39.0	16.0	23.0	10.1	271 000	–	–
Foot	r	990	20.0	6.0	14.0	6.0	36 000	–	–
	l	1 000	20.0	6.0	14.0	6.2	38 000	–	–
Whole body		58 500	165.0						

These data are sufficient for deducing the radii and moments of inertia about any axis through the centre of gravity

According to the rule given on p. 14, as long as the axis of the joint is at right angles to the plane determined by the three points S_1, K, S_2, the moment of inertia of the thigh about the the axis through S_0 and parallel to the axis of the joint is:

$$m_1\left[\varkappa_1^2 + \left(\frac{m_2}{m_1 + m_2}d\right)^2\right]$$

and the moment of inertia of the lower leg + foot system about the axis through S_0 is:

22

Table 3. Ratio of the radius of inertia $\varkappa_0$ to the length of the body segments

Body segments	$\dfrac{\varkappa_0}{l}$	
	Right	Left
Trunk + head	0.23	
Arm	0.27	0.27
Forearm + hand	0.26	0.28
Thigh	0.26	0.27
Lower leg + foot	0.32	0.32
Lower leg	0.25	0.26
Foot	0.30	0.31

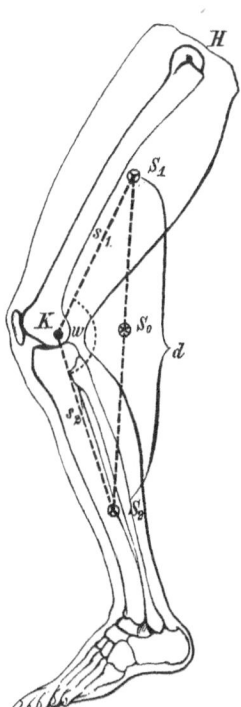

Fig. 3. Finding the moment of inertia of a system of two body segments about an axis through the centre of gravity of this system

$$m_2 \left[\varkappa_2^2 + \left(\frac{m_1}{m_1 + m_2} d \right)^2 \right]$$

$\varkappa_0$ is the radius of inertia of the whole extremity about the axis through the total centre of gravity S_0 and parallel to the axis of the joint. The moment of inertia of the whole extremity is $(m_1 + m_2) \varkappa_0^2$.

23

The following equation pertains:

$$(m_1 + m_2) \varkappa_0^2 = m_1 \left[\varkappa_1^2 + \left(\frac{m_2}{m_1 + m_2} d \right)^2 \right] + m_2 \left[\varkappa_2^2 + \left(\frac{m_1}{m_1 + m_2} d \right)^2 \right].$$

Thus the moment of inertia of a system of bodies is equal to the sum of the moments of inertia of the individual bodies about the same axis.

Transformation of the equation gives:

$$(m_1 + m_2) \varkappa_0^2 = m_1 \varkappa_1^2 + m_2 \varkappa_2^2 + \frac{m_1 m_2}{m_1 + m_2} d^2.$$

This means that:

The moment of inertia of a system of two bodies about any axis through its centre of gravity is equal to the sum of 1. the moments of inertia of the two bodies about the parallel axes through their own centres of gravity and 2. the product of the masses $\dfrac{m_1 m_2}{m_1 + m_2}$ and the square of the distance between the two partial centres of gravity.

Consequently, the moment of inertia of a system of bodies about an axis through its centre of gravity is always greater than the sum of the moments of inertia of the individual parts about parallel axes through their own centres of gravity.

Entering the value of d^2 in the equation above gives:

$$(m_1 + m_2) \varkappa_0^2 = m_1 \varkappa_1^2 + m_2 \varkappa_2^2 + \frac{m_1 m_2}{m_1 + m_2} (s_1^2 + s_2^2 - 2 s_1 s_2 \cos \omega).$$

Except for $\varkappa_0$ and ω, the magnitudes are constant in this equation. Thus they can be used to calculate the radius and moment of inertia of the whole extremity for any degree of flexion:

$$\varkappa_0 = \sqrt{\frac{m_1}{m_1 + m_2} \varkappa_1^2 + \frac{m_2}{m_1 + m_2} \varkappa_2^2 + \frac{m_1 m_2}{(m_1 + m_2)^2} (s_1^2 + s_2^2 - 2 s_1 s_2 \cos \omega)}.$$

During the oscillations of the upper and lower extremities, the elbow and the knee were almost straight. Angle ω in such instances was thus about 180°. Since $\cos 180° = -1$, in this instance the equation for calculating $\varkappa_0$ becomes:

$$\varkappa_0 = \sqrt{\frac{m_1}{m_1 + m_2}\varkappa_1^2 + \frac{m_2}{m_1 + m_2}\varkappa_2^2 + \frac{m_1 m_2}{(m_1 + m_2)^2}(s_1 + s_2)^2}.$$

For the right lower extremity:

$m_1 = 6450$ $m_2 = 3680$

$\varkappa_1 = 10.3$ $\varkappa_2 = 15.1$

$s_1 = 22.3$ $s_2 = 25.0.$

Consequently $\varkappa_0 = 25.6$ cm. Entering the values of the period of the oscillation $\tau = 0.714$ and of the distance between the axis and the centre of gravity of the whole extremity $e = 35.0$ (Table 1) into the equation on p. 14 gives $\varkappa_0 = 23.4$ cm. Actually there is a difference of more than 2 cm between the value of the radius of inertia obtained by direct measurement of the period of oscillation of the whole extremity and that calculated from the moments of inertia of its two segments.

Although this difference is not great, much closer correspondence was to be expected if the main source of error in the first series of experiments could be disposed of.

To avoid interference of any extraneous moments of inertia, in the experiment described so far the axis was either a steel needle or two opposite steel spikes and was fixed to the surroundings. Consequently, the body segment had to oscillate about this fixed steel axis. Obviously friction between the tissues of the oscillating body segment and the steel axis must have exerted a certain influence on the period of oscillation and blurred the results.

Second Series of Experiments

In a second series of experiments we eliminated the source of error by fixing the steel axis to the oscillating body. To this end thicker rods were used with square cross sections. This ensured solid fixation of the steel axis to the body segment. The edge of the steel rod the closest to the centre of gravity of the body segment was used as the axis of oscillation by putting the rod over two thin rods of glass at right angles to it. Hereby friction was reduced to a minimum during oscillation. Actually, once started, the body segment kept oscillating for hours.

In order to determine the distance between the centre of gravity and the axis of oscillation better than by direct measurement, the body segments were all suspended successively from two parallel axes in the plane in which the centre of gravity lay. The two steel rods were both fixed to the body segment before the oscillation with few exceptions. This offered the advantage of placing the rods parallel to each other more accurately and of enabling a check to be made of the solidity of their fixation in relation to each other and to the body segment. Moreover, the distance between the two rods could be measured much more precisely than in the first series of experiments. This method, however, presented the disadvantage that the moments of inertia of the two rods influenced the period of oscillation. Consequently, calculation of the radius of inertia had to eliminate these moments of inertia extraneous to that of the body segment and thus became more complicated. This drawback, however, could not deter us from taking advantage of the greater precision of the results which could be expected from this modification of the method.

The necessary equations are deduced as follows. Figure 4 represents such a steel prism. Its length actually was of course greater in relation to its thickness than Fig. 4 shows. The cross section of the prism is a square with side a and its mass is μ. Its moment of inertia about the longitudinal axis through the centre of gravity is $\mu\dfrac{a^2}{6}$ if the rod is homogeneous or $\mu\dfrac{\delta^2}{3}$ if, rather than a, the half diagonal δ is used since $a^2 = 2\delta^2$.

In Fig. 5, S is the centre of gravity of a body segment (not including the weight of the steel rods), ε_1 and ε_2 the distances from S to the edges A_1 and A_2 closest to S of the two rods. These edges are used as axes of oscillation. They are thicker in Figure 5. The centre of gravity S lies exactly in the plane determined by the two parallel axes A_1 and A_2. The distance between these axes is λ. Therefore:

$$\varepsilon_1 + \varepsilon_2 = \lambda$$

m designates the mass of the body segment without the steel rods,
$\varkappa_0$ the radius of inertia of the body segment only, about the axis A_0
    through its centre of gravity S and parallel to A_1 and A_2,
μ_1 the mass of the steel rod with axis A_1,
δ_1 half the diagonal of its cross section,

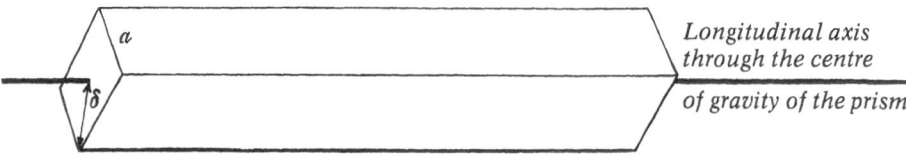

Fig. 4. Steel prism used for suspension of the body segments

μ_2 the mass of the other steel rod with axis A_2,

δ_2 half the diagonal of its cross section,

τ_1 the period of oscillation of the body segment and steel rods system about the axis A_1 for a small amplitude of the oscillation,

τ_2 the corresponding period of oscillation about the axis A_2,

γ the acceleration of gravity.

The moment of inertia of the body segment only, about axis A_1, is:

$$m(\varkappa_0^2 + \varepsilon_1^2).$$

The moment of inertia of the upper steel rod is:

$$\mu_1 \left(\frac{\delta_1^2}{3} + \delta_1^2 \right) = \tfrac{4}{3} \mu_1 \delta_1^2$$

and that of the lower steel rod:

$$\mu_2 \left(\frac{\delta_2^2}{3} + (\lambda + \delta_2)^2 \right) = \tfrac{1}{3} \mu_2 [\delta_2^2 + 3(\lambda + \delta_2)^2].$$

The moment of inertia of the body segment only, about axis A_2, is:

$$m(\varkappa_0^2 + \varepsilon_2^2).$$

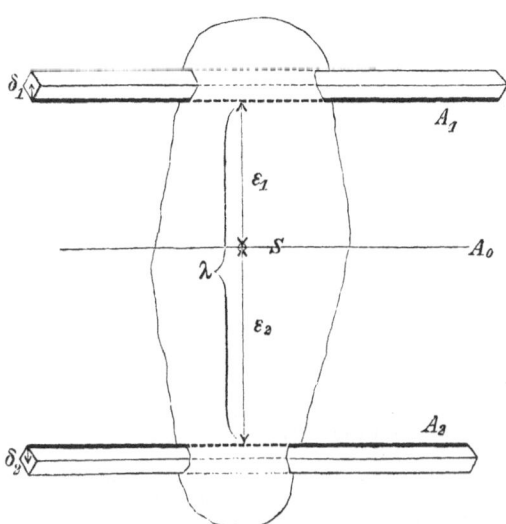

Fig. 5. A body segment with the two parallel steel prisms

The moment of inertia of the upper rod is:

$$\mu_1 \left(\frac{\delta_1^2}{3} + (\lambda + \delta_1)^2 \right) = \tfrac{1}{3} \mu_1 [\delta_1^2 + 3(\lambda + \delta_1)^2]$$

and that of the lower steel rod:

$$\mu_2 \left(\frac{\delta_2^2}{3} + \delta_2^2 \right) = \tfrac{4}{3} \mu_2 \delta_2^2.$$

According to the laws of the pendulum:

$$\tau_1 = \pi \sqrt{\frac{m(\varkappa_0^2 + \varepsilon_1^2) + \tfrac{4}{3}\mu_1 \delta_1^2 + \tfrac{1}{3}\mu_2 [\delta_2^2 + 3(\lambda + \delta_2)^2]}{g[m\varepsilon_1 + \mu_1 \delta_1 + \mu_2(\lambda + \delta_2)]}}$$

$$\tau_2 = \pi \sqrt{\frac{m(\varkappa_0^2 + \varepsilon_2^2) + \tfrac{1}{3}\mu_1 [\delta_1^2 + 3(\lambda + \delta_1)^2] + \tfrac{4}{3}\mu_2 \delta_2^2}{g[m\varepsilon_2 + \mu_1(\lambda + \delta_1) + \mu_2 \delta_2]}}$$

since the period of oscillation of a physical pendulum is $\pi \sqrt{\dfrac{T}{gD}}$ if the amplitude of oscillation is very small. In this equation T is the sum of all the moments of inertia and D the sum of the products of all the small masses and their distance from the axis of oscillation. From these two equations and from equation

$$\varepsilon_1 + \varepsilon_2 = \lambda$$

it results that:

$$\varepsilon_1 = \frac{\lambda[m(\pi^2 \lambda - g\tau_2^2) + g(\mu_2 \tau_1^2 - \mu_1 \tau_2^2) + 2\pi^2(\mu_1 \delta_1 - \mu_2 \delta_2) + \pi^2 \lambda(\mu_1 - \mu_2)] + g(\tau_1^2 - \tau_2^2)(\mu_1 \delta_1 + \mu_2 \delta_2)}{m[2\pi^2 \lambda - g(\tau_1^2 + \tau_2^2)]}$$

$$\varepsilon_2 = \frac{\lambda[m(\pi^2 \lambda - g\tau_1^2) + g(\mu_1 \tau_2^2 - \mu_2 \tau_1^2) + 2\pi^2(\mu_2 \delta_2 - \mu_1 \delta_1) + \pi^2 \lambda(\mu_2 - \mu_1)] + g(\tau_2^2 - \tau_1^2)(\mu_2 \delta_2 + \mu_1 \delta_1)}{m[2\pi^2 \lambda - g(\tau_2^2 + \tau_1^2)]}$$

After ε_1 and ε_2, the radius of inertia $\varkappa_0$ of the body segment only, about the axis A_0 through the centre of gravity, is calculated:

$$\varkappa_0 = \frac{1}{\pi\sqrt{m}} \sqrt{m\varepsilon_1(g\tau_1^2 - \pi^2 \varepsilon_1) + g\tau_1^2(\mu_1 \delta_1 + \mu_2 \delta_2 + \mu_2 \lambda) - \pi^2 [\tfrac{4}{3}(\mu_1 \delta_1^2 + \mu_2 \delta_2^2) + \mu_2 \lambda(2\delta_2 + \lambda)]}$$

This is checked by:

$$\varkappa_0 = \frac{1}{\pi\sqrt{m}} \sqrt{m\varepsilon_2(g\tau_2^2 - \pi^2 \varepsilon_2) + g\tau_2^2(\mu_2 \delta_2 + \mu_1 \delta_1 + \mu_1 \lambda) - \pi^2 [\tfrac{4}{3}(\mu_2 \delta_2^2 + \mu_1 \delta_1^2) + \mu_1 \lambda(2\delta_1 + \lambda)]}$$

In some instances, only one steel rod was present during the oscillation about an edge of this rod. Then the equations were simpler:

$$\tau_1 = \pi \sqrt{\frac{m(\varkappa_0^2 + \varepsilon_1^2) + \frac{4}{3}\mu_1 \delta_1^2}{g(m e_1 + \mu_1 \delta_1)}}$$

$$\tau_2 = \pi \sqrt{\frac{m(\varkappa_0^2 + \varepsilon_2^2) + \frac{4}{3}\mu_2 \delta_2^2}{g(m e_2 + \mu_2 \delta_2)}}$$

$$\varepsilon_1 + \varepsilon_2 = \lambda.$$

Consequently:

$$\varepsilon_1 = \frac{m\lambda(\pi^2 \lambda - g\tau_2^2) + g(\tau_1^2 \mu_1 \delta_1 - \tau_2^2 \mu_2 \delta_2) - \frac{4}{3}\pi^2(\mu_1 \delta_1^2 - \mu_2 \delta_2^2)}{m[2\pi^2 \lambda - g(\tau_1^2 + \tau_2^2)]}$$

$$\varepsilon_2 = \frac{m\lambda(\pi^2 \lambda - g\tau_1^2) + g(\tau_2^2 \mu_2 \delta_2 - \tau_1^2 \mu_1 \delta_1) - \frac{4}{3}\pi^2(\mu_2 \delta_2^2 - \mu_1 \delta_1^2)}{m[2\pi^2 \lambda - g(\tau_2^2 + \tau_1^2)]}$$

and the radius of inertia is:

$$\varkappa_0 = \frac{1}{\pi\sqrt{m}}\sqrt{m\varepsilon_1(g\tau_1^2 - \pi^2 \varepsilon_1) + g\tau_1^2 \mu_1 \delta_1 - \frac{4}{3}\pi^2 \mu_1 \delta_1^2}.$$

This is checked by:

$$\varkappa_0 = \frac{1}{\pi\sqrt{m}}\sqrt{m\varepsilon_2(g\tau_2^2 - \pi^2 \varepsilon_2) + g\tau_2^2 \mu_2 \delta_2 - \frac{4}{3}\pi^2 \mu_2 \delta_2^2}.$$

The second series of experiments were thus carried out as follows. A normally built fairly muscular man hanged himself. The abdomen was not protruding. The cadaver was frozen stiff as for the first series of experiments. The upper and lower extremities were separated from the trunk with the help of saw and knife. The humeral and femoral heads were kept intact and disarticulated. Oscillations were then carried out as follows:

Oscillations of the Trunk and Head System

A steel rod with square cross section was passed through the sockets parallel to the line connecting the centres of the hip joints. The edge of the rod which was to be used as the axis of oscillation A_2 was the

29

closest to the centre of gravity of the trunk and head. A second rod parallel to the first was passed through the neck. The edge of this rod which was to be used as the axis of oscillation A_1 was the closest to the centre of gravity. The centre of gravity lay in the plane determined by the two parallel axes A_1 and A_2.

The dimensions of the steel rods involved in the calculation were: for the upper steel rod with the axis A_1 (through the neck).

Weight   Length of the half diagonal of the cross section
$\mu_1 = 720$ g $\delta_1 = 0.75$ cm

for the lower steel rod with the axis A_2 (through the hip joints)

$\mu_2 = 560$ g $\delta_2 = 0.75$ cm.

The two axes A_1 and A_2 were at a distance $\lambda = 48.75$ cm from each other. The axes were not through the centres of the joints as in series I experiments. Axis A_1 was 7 cm vertical below the centre of the occipito-atlantal joint. Axis A_2 was 1 cm vertically above the line connecting the centres of the two hip joints.

The weight of trunk + head was $m = 23\ 790$ g,
200 pendulum oscillations about the axis A_1 lasted 131.0 s,
200 pendulum oscillations about the axis A_2 134.0 s.

The periods of oscillation thus were: $\tau_1 = 0.655$ s and $\tau_2 = 0.670$ s.

Oscillations of the Trunk Without the Head

The head was sawn along the strangulation furrow. The steel rod was displaced somewhat distally from where it was for the oscillations of the trunk + head. Otherwise there would not have been enough neck and the centre of gravity of the trunk alone would not have been exactly in the plane of the two axes. Consequently, the distance between the two axes was $\lambda = 48.1$ cm and the distance between the axis A_1 and the center of the occipito-atlantal joint 7.65 cm. The length of axis A_2 and the rods were the same as previously.

The weight of the trunk was $m = 19\ 910$ g,
200 oscillations about A_1 lasted 123.4 s,
200 oscillations about A_2 119.6 s.

The period of an oscillation was $\tau_1 = 0.617$ s and $\tau_2 = 0.598$ s.

30

Oscillations of the Head

The head being straight, the two axes were parallel to the line connecting the centres of the hip joints and the centre of gravity of the body segment under consideration, i.e. the head, was in the plane which they determined. This was the case in all experiments and will not be repeated.

The upper axis A_1 was close to the vertex, the lower A_2 was 2 cm on a vertical line below the occipito-atlantal joint. The distance between the two axes was $\lambda = 16.6$ cm. The steel rods were thinner than previously. For the upper steel rod with the axis A_1: $\mu_1 = 105$ g, $\delta_1 = 0.3$ cm; for the lower with the axis A_2: $\mu_2 = 140$ g, $\delta_2 = 0.4$ cm.

The head weighed $m = 3880$ g,
200 oscillations about A_1 lasted 77.8 s,
200 oscillations about A_2 74.8 s.

Consequently: $\tau_1 = 0.389$ s and $\tau_2 = 0.374$ s.

Oscillations of the Left Leg

The upper axis A_1 had the same direction as the line connecting the centres of the hip joints when the leg was extended and thus was at right angles to the longitudinal axis. It was 0.6 cm below the centre of the femoral head. The lower axis A_2 was parallel to the first and 2.5 cm above the centre of the ankle. The distance between the two axes was $\lambda = 70.1$ cm.

For the upper steel rod with the axis A_1: $\mu_1 = 151$ g and $\delta_1 = 0.5$ cm; for the lower with the axis A_2: $\mu_2 = 157$ g and $\delta_2 = 0.5$ cm.

The leg weighed $m = 7640$ g,
200 oscillations about A_1 lasted 145.2 s,
200 oscillations about A_2 149.1 s.

Consequently: $\tau_1 = 0.726$ s and $\tau_2 = 0.7455$ s.

Oscillations of the Left Thigh

The thigh was disarticulated at knee level. The two axes were parallel to the axis of the knee. The upper one A_1 was the same as A_1 for the leg. The lower one was 2.7 cm above the axis of the knee. The distance between the two axes was $\lambda = 33.35$ cm.

31

For the upper steel rod with the axis A_1: $\mu_1 = 151$ g and $\delta_2 = 0.5$ cm; for the lower with the axis A_2: $\mu_1 = 59$ g and $\delta_2 = 0.3$ cm.

The thigh weighed $m = 4810$ g,
200 oscillations about A_1 lasted 98.4 s,
200 oscillations about A_2 101.8 s.

Consequently: $\tau_1 = 0.492$ s and $\tau_2 = 0.509$ s.

Oscillations of the Left Lower Leg and Foot System

The axes were also parallel to the axis of the knee. The lower one A_2 was the same as A_2 for the leg whereas the upper one A_1 was 5.3 cm below the axis of the knee. The distance between the two axes was $\lambda = 29.3$ cm.

For the upper steel rod: $\mu_1 = 55.5$ g and $\delta_1 = 0.3$ cm; for the lower: $\mu_2 = 157$ g and $\delta_2 = 0.5$ cm.

The system weighed $m = 2800$ g,
200 oscillations about A_1 lasted 110.4 s,
200 oscillations about A_2 110.9 s.

Consequently: $\tau_1 = 0.552$ s and $\tau_2 = 0.5545$ s.

Oscillations of the Left Lower Leg

The two axes were the same as for the lower leg + foot system. The centre of gravity of the lower leg only was a little behind the plane determined by A_1 and A_2 since in the previous experiment this plane comprised the centre of gravity of the lower leg + foot system. This source of error, however, had little effect on the result since the sum of the distances from the centre of gravity of the lower leg to the two axes is very little different from the direct distance between the two axes. The magnitude λ is the only one to be modified by the position of the centre of gravity outside the plane determined by the axes A_1 and A_2.

The lower leg weighed 1890 g,
200 oscillations about A_1 lasted 92.7 s, and
200 oscillations about A_2 97.5 s.

Consequently: $\tau_1 = 0.4635$ s and $\tau_2 = 0.4875$ s.

Oscillations of the Left Foot

The upper axis A_1 was parallel to the axis of the ankle joint, 1 cm lower and somewhat more anterior so that it was in the plane determined by the axis of the ankle joint and the centre of gravity of the foot. The lower axis A_2 was in the same plane, parallel to the first axis and at a distance $\lambda = 7.55$ cm from it.

For the upper steel rod $\mu_1 = 56$ g and $\delta_1 = 0.3$ cm; for the lower, $\mu_2 = 74$ g and $\delta_2 = 0.4$ cm.

The foot weighed 910 g,
200 oscillations about A_1 lasted 68.1 s,
200 oscillations about A_2 89.4 s.

Consequently: $\tau_1 = 0.3405$ s and $\tau_2 = 0.447$ s.

Oscillations of the Left Thigh About Axes Parallel to Its Longitudinal Axis

The two parallel axes were at a distance $\lambda = 5.5$ cm from each other. For the steel rod with the axis A_1: $\mu_1 = 231.5$ g and $\delta_1 = 0.5$ cm; for the other with the axis A_2: $\mu_2 = 98.5$ cm and $\delta_2 = 0.4$ cm. The plane determined by the axes A_1 and A_2 comprised the centre of gravity of the thigh and, within a close approximation, its longitudinal axis, i.e. the line connecting the centres of the two adjacent joints[4]. In this instance, each of the steel rods consisted of two parts, one in the hip end and the other in the knee end. Both of these parts were aligned as accurately as possible. The same arrangement was used in all experiments of oscillations about axes parallel to the longitudinal axis of a body segment.

200 oscillations about the axis A_1 lasted 60.5 s,
200 oscillations about the axis A_2 118.2 s.

Consequently: $\tau_1 = 0.3025$ s and $\tau_2 = 0.591$ s.

During these oscillations only one rod was present in the body segment.

---

[4] Braune W, Fischer O (1984) On the centre of gravity of the human body. Springer, Berlin Heidelberg New York Tokyo.

Oscillations of the Left Lower Leg About Axes Parallel to Its Longitudinal Axis

The two parallel axes were at a distance $\lambda = 3.2$ cm from each other. For one steel rod $\mu_1 = 98.5$ g and $\delta_1 = 0.4$ cm; for the other $\mu_2 = 165.5$ g and $\delta_2 = 0.5$ cm.

The plane determined by the two axes comprised the centre of gravity of the lower leg and its longitudinal axis.

200 oscillations about A_1 lasted 49.8 s,
200 oscillations about A_2 73.0 s.

Consequently: $\tau_1 = 0.249$ s and $\tau_2 = 0.365$ s.

In this experiment also, only one steel rod at a time was present in the body segment, the one which corresponded to the axis of oscillation.

Oscillations of the Left Foot About Vertical Axes

The two axes were parallel to the longitudinal axis of the lower leg with the foot in the neutral position. The distance from each other was $\lambda = 9$ cm.

For the steel rod closer to the lower leg with the axis $A_1: \mu_1 = 49.2$ g and $\delta_1 = 0.4$ cm; for the other with the axis $A_2: \mu_2 = 155.7$ g and $\delta_2 = 0.75$ cm. Here also the centre of gravity of the foot was in the plane determined by A_1 and A_2.

200 oscillations about A_1 lasted 700 s,
200 oscillations about A_2 71.0 s.

Consequently: $\tau_1 = 0.350$ s and $\tau_2 = 0.355$ s.

During this experiment, as in all others except where indicated, both steel rods were present in the body segment during its oscillations.

Oscillations of the Left Arm

The upper axis A_1 had the same direction as the line connecting the centres of the two humeral heads with the arms hanging in neutral position and was at right angles to the longitudinal axis of the humerus. It was 1.8 cm below the centre of the humeral head. The lower axis A_2 was parallel to the first, between the fourth and fifth metacarpals. The distance between the two axes was $\lambda = 52.5$ cm. The centre of gravity of the arm was in the plane determined by the two axes.

For the upper steel rod $\mu_1 = 80.2$ g and $\delta_1 = 0.5$ cm; for the lower $\mu_2 = 49$ g and $\delta_2 = 0.4$ cm.

The arm weighed 2470 g,
200 oscillations about A_1 lasted 123.9 s,
200 oscillations about A_2 125.9 s.

Consequently: $\tau_1 = 0.6195$ s and $\tau_2 = 0.6295$ s.

Oscillations of the Left Upper Arm

The upper axis A_1 was different from A_1 in the previous experiment. It was parallel to the axis of the elbow joint and through the centre of the humeral head. The lower axis A_2 was also parallel to and 1 cm above the axis of the elbow joint. The plane determined by the two axes comprised the centre of gravity of the upper arm. The distance between the two axes was $\lambda = 26.1$ cm.

For the upper steel rod $\mu_1 = 49$ g and $\delta_1 = 0.4$ cm; for the lower $\mu_2 = 85$ g and $\delta_2 = 0.5$ cm.

The upper arm weighed 1 252 g,
200 oscillations about A_1 lasted 86.1 s,
200 oscillations about A_2 86.8 s.

Consequently: $\tau_1 = 0.4305$ s and $\tau_2 = 0.434$ s.

Oscillations of the Forearm and Hand System

The upper axis A_1 was parallel to and 3.5 cm below the axis of the elbow joint. The lower axis A_2 was parallel to and at a distance $\lambda = 26.0$ cm from the upper one. The plane determined by A_1 and A_2 comprised the centre of gravity of the forearm + hand system.

For the upper steel rod $\mu_1 = 54.7$ g and $\delta_1 = 0.4$ cm; for the lower $\mu_2 = 49.2$ g and $\delta_2 = 0.4$ cm.

The system weighed 1 205 g,
200 oscillations about A_1 lasted 96.4 s,
200 oscillations about A_2 96.0 s.

Consequently: $\tau_1 = 0.482$ s and $\tau_2 = 0.480$ s.

Oscillations of the Left Upper Arm About Axes Parallel to Its Longitudinal Axis

The two parallel axes determined a plane in which the centre of gravity lay and were at a distance $\lambda = 4.0$ cm from each other.

For one steel rod $\mu_1 = 38$ g and $\delta_1 = 0.3$ cm ; for the other $\mu_2 = 78$ g and $\delta_2 = 0.4$ cm.

Here also, as in the experiment on oscillations of the left thigh about axes parallel to its longitudinal axis, each of the two rods was made of two parts, one as the continuation of the other.

200 oscillations about A_1 lasted 47.4 s,
200 oscillations about A_2 48.9 s.

Consequently: $\tau_1 = 0.237$ s and $\tau_2 = 0.2445$ s.

Oscillations of the Forearm and Hand System About Axes Parallel to Its Longitudinal Axis

The two parallel axes were at a distance $\lambda = 4.5$ cm from each other.

For one steel rod $\mu_1 = 165.2$ g and $\delta_1 = 0.5$ cm; for the other $\mu_2 = 104$ g and $\delta_2 = 0.4$ cm.

The plane determined by the two axes comprised the centre of gravity of the forearm + hand system and the longitudinal axis of the forearm, with the hand in the neutral position.

200 oscillations about A_1 lasted 46.2 s,
200 oscillations about A_2 47.6 s.

Consequently: $\tau_1 = 0.231$ s and $\tau_2 = 0.238$ s.

The corresponding oscillation experiments were then carried out for the right limbs. The 13 groups of measurements follow each other exactly in the same order as for the left limbs. There is thus no need to give their description in detail. The values of $\lambda, \mu_1, \mu_2, \delta_1, \delta_2, \tau_1$ and τ_2 resulting from our measurements are shown in Tables 4 and 5. It must be mentioned that, during the oscillations of the right arm, the steel rod with the axis A_2 was not through the hand as on the left side but through the ulna because it could no longer be fixed solidly in the hand. In the course of the experiments, the soft parts in the vicinity of the hand were no longer frozen so hard that any flexion of the wrist could be reliably excluded during the oscillations when the steel rod was through the hand. The elbow joint remained sufficiently frozen.

Table 4. Data necessary for calculation of the moments of inertia about axes at right angles to the longitudinal axis of the body segments (second series of experiments)

Body segments		m	μ_1	δ_1	μ_2	δ_2	λ	τ_1	τ_2
Trunk + head		23 790	720.0	0.75	560.0	0.75	48.75	0.655	0.670
Trunk		19 910	720.0	0.75	560.0	0.75	48.1	0.617	0.598
Head		3 880	105.0	0.3	140.0	0.4	16.6	0.389	0.374
Leg	r	7 840	155.5	0.5	139.0	0.5	70.9	0.728	0.7455
	l	7 640	151.0	0.5	157.0	0.5	70.1	0.726	0.7455
Thigh	r	4 860	155.5	0.5	151.0	0.5	35.1	0.4995	0.513
	l	4 810	151.0	0.5	59.0	0.3	33.35	0.492	0.509
Lower leg + foot	r	2 980	144.5	0.5	139.0	0.5	31.2	0.560	0.5575
	l	2 800	55.5	0.3	157.0	0.5	29.3	0.552	0.5545
Lower leg	r	2 070	144.5	0.5	139.0	0.5	31.2	0.457	0.499
	l	1 890	55.5	0.3	157.0	0.5	29.3	0.4635	0.4875
Foot	r	910	54.7	0.4	80.2	0.5	10.1	0.3445	0.3425
	l	910	56.0	0.3	74.0	0.4	7.55	0.3405	0.447
Arm	r	2 360	85.0	0.5	54.7	0.4	38.1	0.6135	0.612
	l	2 470	80.2	0.5	49.0	0.4	52.5	0.6195	0.6295
Upper arm	r	1 243	55.7	0.3	80.5	0.5	25.0	0.4255	0.4345
	l	1 252	49.0	0.4	85.0	0.5	26.1	0.4305	0.434
Forearm + hand	r	1 117	49.5	0.4	54.8	0.4	25.2	0.467	0.465
	l	1 205	54.7	0.4	49.2	0.4	26.0	0.482	0.480

The unit of mass is the gram, that of length the centimetre and that of time the second

Table 5. Data necessary for calculation of the moments of inertia about the long axis of the body segments (second series of experiments)

Body segments		m	μ_1	δ_1	μ_2	δ_2	λ	τ_1	τ_2
Thigh	r	4860	114.7	0.5	219.2	0.5	5.1	0.403	0.305
	l	4810	231.5	0.5	98.5	0.4	5.5	0.3025	0.591
Lower leg	r	2070	114.7	0.5	112.1	0.4	4.4	0.250	0.2755
	l	1890	98.5	0.4	165.5	0.5	3.2	0.249	0.365
Foot	r	910	49.2	0.4	80.3	0.5	9.2	0.353	0.3555
	l	910	49.2	0.4	155.7	0.75	9.0	0.350	0.355
Upper arm	r	1243	69.5	0.4	134.7	0.4	4.5	0.236	0.246
	l	1252	38.0	0.3	78.0	0.4	4.0	0.237	0.2445
Forearm + hand	r	1117	75.1	0.4	106.7	0.4	2.1	0.2775	0.2915
	l	1205	165.2	0.5	104.0	0.4	4.5	0.231	0.238

The units are grams, centimetres, and seconds

Therefore, λ is significantly smaller in this experiment than in its counterpart on the left side. For the same reason the distance between the two axes during the oscillations of the right forearm + hand system about an axis parallel to its longitudinal axis is shorter than on the left side. In this instance the two steel rods had to be placed in bone to secure solid fixation to the body segment.

Only the data necessary for the calculation of the moments of inertia and resulting from direct measurements are shown in Tables 4 and 5.

In these experiments, during the oscillations, both steel rods were fixed in the body segment. Therefore, the equations on p. 28 can be used to calculate the distances ε_1 and ε_2 between the centre of gravity and the axes, and the radius of inertia $\varkappa_0$. In the tables the data concerning the foot do not relate to the axes at right angles to the longitudinal axis of the foot but to axes at right angles to the longitudinal axis of the lower leg with the foot in the neutral position.

During the oscillations of the foot mentioned in Table 5 the two axes were not parallel to the longitudinal axis of the foot but parallel to the longitudinal axis of the lower leg, the foot being in the neutral position. The position of the two steel rods was such that the equations on p. 28 could also be used. During all the other oscillations, the results of which are given in Table 5, only the steel rod with the axis was present in the body segment. Therefore, for these oscillations about axes parallel to the longitudinal axis of the body segment the other equations on p. 29 must be used.

The acceleration of gravity in Leipzig $g = 981.11$ was used in all the calculations in the second series of experiments.

The equations on pp. 28 and 29 enabled the distances ε_1 and ε_2 between the centre of gravity of each body segment and the axes of oscillation to be calculated from the data in Table 4. The results are given in Table 6 [5].

For the right lower leg + foot system the distance between the two axes of oscillation and the positions of the axes were fortuitously such that the expression $\pi^2 \lambda - g \tau_1^2$ in the second equation was very small. Consequently, a small error in the magnitudes λ and τ_1 had considerable consequences for the result. Therefore, the directly measured magnitudes could not be used to calculate the distances between the centre of gravity and the axes, and the radius of inertia. It will be shown later how in this instance an acceptable value of the radius of inertia can be obtained through a roundabout way.

---

[5] Dr. Höckner, assistant at the Office of the Leipziger Stadtvermessung, kindly calculated these values for us as well as those of ε_1 and ε_2 given in Table 8 and those of $\varkappa_0$ given in Table 9. To this end he applied the equations on pp. 28 and 29 and used a calculator.

Table 6. Distances ε_1 and ε_2 between the centre of gravity and the axes of oscillation at right angles to the longitudinal axis of the body segment

Body segments	ε_1		ε_2	
	Right	Left	Right	Left
Trunk + head	19.61		29.14	
Trunk	26.85		21.25	
Head	10.53		6.07	
Leg	32.74	31.82	38.16	38.28
Thigh	15.72	15.30	19.38	18.05
Lower leg + foot	–	16.64	–	12.66
Lower leg	11.43	11.00	19.77	18.30
Foot	4.78	5.95	5.32	1.60
Arm	22.18	25.37	15.92	27.13
Upper arm	11.37	12.31	13.63	13.79
Forearm + hand	12.89	13.52	12.31	12.48

The magnitudes ε_1 and ε_2 express the distances between the centre of gravity and the axes of oscillation which were chosen arbitrarily. They are not actually the distances between the centre of gravity and the centres of the adjacent joints since in the second series of experiments the axes did not pass through the centres of the joints. Therefore, no conclusion can be drawn as yet from the values of ε_1 and ε_2. If in some instances these values are about the same for the two sides of the body, this finally results from a generally symmetrical placement of the axes on both sides of the body.

To obtain the distances e_1 and e_2 between the centre of gravity and the centres of the adjacent joints, the magnitudes ε_1 and ε_2 must be increased by the distances a_1 and a_2 between the axes A_1 and A_2 and the adjacent centres of the joints. These distances have been measured in every experiment (Table 7).

The distances e between the centre of gravity and the centres of the adjacent joints were obtained by adding ε to a. They are given in Table 9.

The equations on p. 29 enable the distances ε_1 and ε_2 between the axes of oscillation and the centre of gravity on the longitudinal axis of the body segment to be calculated from the oscillations about axes parallel to the longitudinal axis. For the oscillations of the foot the equations on pp. 28 and 29 must be used (Table 8).

These values cannot be used as such, since the positions of the axes of oscillation were chosen arbitrarily. However, they had to be calculated because they enable the radius of inertia about the longitudinal axis of the body segment to be deduced.

Table 7. Distances a_1 and a_2 between the axes A_1 and A_2 and the adjacent centres of the joints

Body segments	a_1		a_2	
	Right	Left	Right	Left
Trunk + head	23.0		1.0	
Trunk	7.65		1.0	
Head	1.4		− 2.0[a]	
Leg	0	0.6	8.0	8.5
Thigh	0	0.6	0.8	2.7
Lower leg + foot	4.7	5.3	8.0	8.5
Lower leg	4.7	5.3	2.0	2.5
Foot	1.6	1.0	−	−
Arm	3.0	1.8	−	−
Upper arm	0	0	0.5	1.0
Forearm + hand	3.1	3.5	−	−

[a] This distance is negative because the axis A_2 was below the occipito-atlantal joint during the oscillation of the head

Table 8. Distances ε_1 and ε_2 between the centre of gravity and the axes of oscillation parallel to the longitudinal axis of the body segment

Body segments	ε_1		ε_2	
	Right	Left	Right	Left
Thigh	1.39	4.90	3.71	0.60
Lower leg	2.79	2.50	1.61	0.70
Foot	4.65	4.55	4.55	4.45
Upper arm	2.72	2.23	1.78	1.77
Forearm + hand	1.13	2.54	0.97	1.96

The radius of inertia $\varkappa_0$ about axes through the centre of gravity of the body segment and at right angles to its longitudinal axis is calculated using the two equations on p. 28, which confirm each other. The same equations are used to calculate the radii of inertia about the two axes through the centre of gravity of the foot. One of these axes is at right angles and the other is parallel to the longitudinal axis of the lower leg when the foot is in the neutral position. The radii of inertia about the longitudinal axes of the different body segments are calculated using the two equations for $\varkappa_0$ on p. 29. These two equations confirm each other.

Table 9 gives the calculated values of $\varkappa_0^2$, those of the moment of inertia $m \varkappa_0^2$, the distances between the centre of gravity of the body segment and the centres of the adjacent joints, the length of each body segment, i.e. the distance between the centres of the adjacent joints, and the mass of each body segment. Although in most instances only the moments of inertia about two axes of the same body segment were deduced, Table 9 gives all the data which characterize the different body segments mechanically. This will appear in further discussion.

Before drawing conclusions from these results, examination of the instances in which the moments of inertia have been calculated for a system of body segments as well as for its different parts will show that the second series of experiments gave much more precise results than did the first.

$\varkappa_1$ and $\varkappa_2$ are the radii of inertia of two articulated body segments about two axes through their centres of gravity and parallel to the axis of the joint when the latter is a hinge joint. m_1 and m_2 are the masses of the body segments. s_1 and s_2 are the distances between the centres of gravity of the two body segments and the axis of the joint. $\varkappa_0$ is the radius of inertia of the system comprising the two body segments about an axis through its centre of gravity and parallel to the axis of the joint. ω is the angle of flexion. According to the discussion on p. 24, the following equation pertains:

$$(m_1 + m_2)\varkappa_0^2 = m_1 \varkappa_1^2 + m_2 \varkappa_2^2 + \frac{m_1 m_2}{m_1 + m_2}(s_1^2 + s_2^2 - 2 s_1 s_2 \cos \omega).$$

Except for the lower leg + foot system, the angle of flexion ω was about 180° for all the systems on which we carried out the oscillation experiments. Therefore (see p. 24):

$$(m_1 + m_2)\varkappa_0^2 = m_1 \varkappa_1^2 + m_2 \varkappa_2^2 + \frac{m_1 m_2}{m_1 + m_2}(s_1 + s_2)^2.$$

If, in every instance, an index 1 is added to the magnitudes m, s and $\varkappa$ of the proximal body segment and an index 2 to those of the distal body segment, s_1 corresponds to the magnitude designated as e_2 in Table 9 and s_2 to that designated as e_1.

Thus calculated $\varkappa_0$ is for

the trunk + head	21.09		21.08
the left leg	24.30	whereas direct	25.08
the right arm	17.63	measurement gave	18.38
the left arm	18.59		17.60.

Table 9. Masses, positions of the centres of gravity and moments of inertia of the body segments (second series of experiments)

Body segments		Mass m (g)	Length l (cm)	Distance between centre of gravity and centre of joint (cm)		Radius of inertia x_0 and moment of inertia $T = m x_0^2$ about axes through the centre of gravity			
						Axes at right angles to the longitudinal axis of the body segment		Longitudinal axis of the body segment	
				e_1 Above	e_2 Below	x_0 (cm)	T (cm² g)	x_0 (cm)	T (cm² g)
Trunk + head		23 790	72.75	42.61	30.14	21.08	10 571 500	—	—
Trunk	r	19 910	56.75ª	34.50	22.25	16.73	5 574 600	—	—
Head		3 880	16.0ᵇ	11.93	4.07	6.81	179 940	—	—
Leg	r	7 840	78.9	32.74	46.16	25.10	4 939 300	—	—
	l	7 640	79.2	32.42	46.78	25.08	4 805 600	—	—
Thigh	r	4 860	35.9	15.72	20.18	11.01	589 100	4.55	100 610
	l	4 810	36.65	15.90	20.75	11.43	628 400	4.56	100 020
Lower leg + foot	r	2 980	43.9	(24.77)ᶠ	(19.13)ᶠ	(14.41)ᶠ	(618 555)ᶠ	—	—
	l	2 800	43.1	21.94	21.16	15.10	638 400	—	—
Lower leg	r	2 070	37.9	16.13	21.77	9.16	173 680	3.12	20 150
	l	1 890	37.1	16.30	20.80	9.66	176 370	3.05	17 580
Foot	r	910	6.0 Height / 20.0ᶜ Length	6.38	13.62	5.91	31 785	6.21	35 093
Foot	l	910	6.0 Height / 20.0ᶜ Length	6.95	13.05	5.97	32 433	6.24	35 433
Arm	r	2 360	59.0	25.18	33.82	18.38	797 300	—	—
	l	2 470	58.5	27.17	31.33	17.60	765 100	—	—

Upper arm {r	1 243	25.5	11.37	14.13	7.95	78 560	2.79	9 680
{l	1 252	27.1	12.31	14.79	7.79	75 980	2.74	9 400
Forearm + hand {r	1 117	36.0[d]	15.99	20.01	10.43	121 500	2.75	8 450
{l	1 205	35.5[e]	17.02	18.48	11.24	152 200	2.71	8 850
Whole body	44 057	150.5						

[a] Length of the trunk means the distance between the centre of the occipito-atlantal joint and the line connecting the centres of the hip joints

[b] Length of the head means the distance between the vertex and the centre of the occipito-atlantal joint

[c] Length of the foot means the distance between the tip of the foot and the ankle joint

[d] This includes 24 cm, the length of the forearm, and 12 cm, the distance between the wrist and the first interphalangeal joint

[e] This includes 25 cm, the length of the forearm, and 10.5 cm, the distance between the wrist and the first interphalangeal joint

[f] These four values were not obtained by direct measurement but through a roundabout way (see p. 44). They thus cannot be as accurate as the others

For the lower leg + foot system ω is not 180° but about 120°. ω is the angle formed by the lines connecting the centres of gravity and the centre of the ankle joint.

Since $\cos 120° = -0.5$, in this instance the general relation is transformed into:

$$(m_1 + m_2)\varkappa_0^2 = m_1\varkappa_1^2 + m_2\varkappa_2^2 + \frac{m_1 m_2}{m_1 + m_2}(s_1^2 + s_1 s_2 + s_2^2).$$

The radius of inertia $\varkappa_0$ thus is, for the right lower leg + foot system: 14.41; for the left lower leg + foot system: 14.55.

Direct measurement gave 15.10 for the left side. There was no measurement for the right side as mentioned above. The value $\varkappa_0 = 14.41$ for the right lower leg + foot system can be entered into the equation on p. 41 together with the values of $\varkappa_0$ directly measured for the right leg and thigh to obtain in a backward way the value of s_2, i.e. the magnitude designated as e_1 in Table 9 (distance between the centre of gravity of the lower leg + foot system and the axis of the knee). It appears that $s_2 = e_1 = 24.77$ and, since $\lambda = 43.9$, $e_2 = 19.13$. The moment of inertia itself is 618 555. These four magnitudes are also given in Table 9.

If the values of the radii of inertia calculated from the moments of inertia of the different body segments are compared with those obtained by direct measurement of the periods of oscillation of the body segments, the relatively small discrepancies demonstrate that the results of the second series of experiments are much more accurate than the results of the first series. The greatest possible accuracy has been attained. By the way it must be noticed that the assumptions $\omega = 180°$ in the former instances and $\omega = 120°$ in the latter are only approximate.

The degree of accuracy is also demonstrated by the fact that the values of the radii of inertia of the body segments on both sides differ only by some millimeters at a maximum in many instances (for example, for the legs and feet). All moments of inertia about the long axis of the body segments differ only by tenths of a millimeter.

Separation of the body segments from each other represented a significant source of error. There was no way of separating the body segments on both sides perfectly symmetrically. Despite this apparently important source of error the magnitudes of the radii of inertia for the body segments on the two sides match each other so well as to enforce the concept that the radius of inertia is a magnitude subjected to very small variations despite relatively large variations in the arrangement of the masses. Consequently, *the variations in the distribu-*

tion of the masses which result from both circulation and muscular contraction exert only a limited influence on the magnitude of the radius of inertia of every body segment.

We found the same behaviour for the position of the centre of gravity of every body segment[6]. The position of the centres of gravity coincided closely not only in the same body segments on both sides of a subject but in all corresponding body segments in our subjects as well as in those of Harless. The variations which the centre of gravity of a body segment is subjected to as a result of the displacements of its masses during muscular contraction or because of blood circulation can be demonstrated. However, they are not sufficient to exert a significant influence on the position of the centre of gravity when the movement of articulated body segments is analysed. Although they appeared very small from our measurements, the individual variations of the position of the centre of gravity are always larger than those resulting from blood circulation and muscular contraction.

The masses, position of the centre of gravity, and moments of inertia of the head, thigh, lower leg, foot, upper arm, forearm and even those of the hand and trunk, but with some more approximation, can be considered as constant. These magnitudes determine the behaviour of any body whatever its form, towards moving forces. The body segments mentioned above thus can be considered as given invariable masses in a purely mechanical sense, i.e. as far as their behaviour towards moving forces is concerned. This makes the mechanics of the human body manageable mathematically and physically. Analysis of the mechanical conditions then deals with a complex of rigid bodies the different parts of which articulate with each other in a well-determined way and are subjected to external and internal forces which can evoke a change in their position in relation one to an other. After this problem is solved, the hypothesis that the parts are absolutely constant can be dismissed and the influence exerted by changes in the different parts, for example movements of the fingers and the phalanges, on the whole body can then be analysed.

The ratio of the radius of inertia x_0 about the axes at right angles to the longitudinal axis of a body segment, to the length l of this body segment is calculated using the data in the third and sixth columns in Table 9. The results are given in Table 10.

---

[6] Braune W, Fischer O (1984) On the centre of gravity of the human body. Springer, Berlin Heidelberg New York Tokyo.

Table 10. Ratio of the radius of inertia $\varkappa_0$ about axes at right angles to the longitudinal axis of a body segment, to the length l of this body segment

Body segments	$\dfrac{\varkappa_0}{l}$	
	Right	Left
Trunk + head	0.29	
Trunk	0.29	
Head	0.43	
Leg	0.32	0.32
Thigh	0.31	0.31
Lower leg + foot	0.33	0.35
Lower leg	0.24	0.26
Foot	0.30	0.30
Arm	0.31	0.30
Upper arm	0.31	0.29
Forearm + hand	0.29	0.32

The length of the head is the distance between the vertex and the centre of the occipito-atlantal joint. If the distance between the vertex and the chin, about 22 cm in our subject, is considered as the length of the head, the ratio $\dfrac{\varkappa_0}{l}$ is 0.31.

This ratio again appears to be about the same for all body segments, as in the first series of experiments. Its average value is 0.30. The average value in the first series was 0.28.

Consequently: *In all segments of the human body the ratio of the radius of inertia about any axis through the centre of gravity of the segment and at right angles to its longitudinal axis, to the length of the segment is always about 0.30.*

The length of a body segment is the distance between the centres of the two adjacent joints, except for the head.

There is no such relationship between the radii of inertia about the longitudinal axis of the body segment and the length of this segment. However, such a relationship exists between this radius of inertia and the average diameter of the body segment, at least for the cases which we have analysed.

We failed to measure the average diameter of the body segments of the cadavers used for our researches. However, it can be assumed that in two similar bodies without undue fat the ratio of the average diameter of a body segment to its length is constant. In our previous work on the centre of gravity of the human body[7] we studied a normal individual without undue fat and sawed its body segments through their centre of gravity perpendicular to their long axis. These cross sections are reproduced in that work.

The average diameter of the thigh was 14.2 cm, that of the upper arm 9.3 cm. Since the two cross sections were carried out through the centre of gravity, their diameter can be considered as the average diameter of the body segment. This would not be true for the lower leg because of its peculiar shape. In this case we took the average of the diameters of the cross sections through the centre of gravity of the lower leg (cross section 8) and through the centre of gravity of the lower leg + foot (cross section 9). This average diameter is 9.8 cm. In this body the thigh was 40.0 cm long, the lower leg 41.5 cm and the upper arm 32.0 cm. In this instance the ratio of the average diameter to the length of the body segment thus was:

0.355 for the thigh
0.235 for the lower leg
0.29 for the upper arm.

In the cadaver used for the present second series of experiments, the lengths of the body segments were as follows (Table 9):

Thigh	R 35.9 cm
	L 36.65 cm
Lower leg	R 37.9 cm
	L 37.1 cm
Upper arm	R 25.5 cm
	L 27.1 cm

Multiplying these lengths and the ratios of the average diameter to the length gives the following data, which have only limited value.

		d
Average diameter of the thigh	R	12.75 cm
	L	13.0 cm
Lower leg	R	8.9 cm
	L	8.7 cm
Upper arm	R	7.4 cm
	L	7.9 cm

[7] Braune W, Fischer O (1984) On the centre of gravity of the human body. Springer, Berlin Heidelberg New York Tokyo, pp. 22, 23.

The radius of inertia about the longitudinal axis of the body segment, as given in Table 9, is as follows:

$$\varkappa_0$$

		$\varkappa_0$
For the thigh	R	4.55 cm
	L	4.56 cm
Lower leg	R	3.12 cm
	L	3.05 cm
Upper arm	R	2.79 cm
	L	2.74 cm

The ratio of the radius of inertia $\varkappa_0$ about the longitudinal axis of the body segment, to its average diameter d is:

		$\dfrac{\varkappa_0}{d}$
For the thigh	R	0.36
	L	0.35
Lower leg	R	0.35
	L	0.35
Upper arm	R	0.38
	L	0.35

It was arbitrarily assumed that the relationship between the average diameter and the length of the body segments was the same in the two cadavers, cadaver IV in the analysis of the centre of gravity and cadaver II in the present series of experiments. However, the ratio of the radius of inertia to the average diameter appears surprisingly constant. In most instances it is 0.35. Unfortunately it was not possible to determine the radius of inertia of the forearm about its longitudinal axis. But the same relationship is to be expected as a consequence of the shape of the forearm. This should be examined when an opportunity occurs. The results can be summarized:

The ratio of the radius of inertia about the longitudinal axis, to the average diameter of the thigh, the lower leg, the upper arm and presumably also the forearm, is constant at about 0.35.

This rule and that on p. 46 enable *the radii and moments of inertia of every body segment about all axes perpendicular to the longitudinal axis and about the longitudinal axis itself to be deduced in vivo with a good degree of approximation.* To this end, only the lengths and average diameters of the body segments need be measured. If l designates the length, d the average diameter, $\varkappa_0'$ the radius of inertia about an axis at right angles to the longitudinal axis and $\varkappa_0''$ the radius of inertia about the longitudinal axis itself, then:

$$\varkappa_0' = 0.3\,l \quad \text{and} \quad \varkappa_0'' = 0.35\,d.$$

To deduce the moment of inertia, the mass of every body segment must be known. Table 9 (p. 42) gives the masses of the subject in our second series of experiments. The ratio μ of the mass of the body segment to the mass of the whole body has been calculated and is given in Table 11.

If the mass of the body, easily measurable in vivo, is M then the mass m of each segment of a body of the same constitution is:

$$m = \mu M.$$

The moment of inertia T'' about an axis through the centre of gravity and at right angles to the longitudinal axis of the body segment is:

$$T' = 0.09\,\mu M\,l^2.$$

The moment of inertia T'' about the longitudinal axis of the body segment is

$$T'' = 0.1225\,\mu M\,d^2$$

μ is taken from Table 11; M, l and d can be measured directly on the living subject.

Table 11. Ratio μ of the mass of a body segment to the mass of the whole body

Body segments	μ		μ
	Right	Left	Average
Head	0.088		0.088
Trunk	0.452		0.452
Thigh	0.110	0.109	0.110
Lower leg	0.047	0.043	0.045
Foot	0.021	0.021	0.021
Upper arm	0.028	0.029	0.028
Forearm + hand	0.027	0.025	0.026
Total	1.000		

Deduction of the Moments of Inertia About Any Axis Through the Centre of Gravity

$\mathcal{T}$he radius of inertia of every body segment about the longitudinal axis and that about an axis through the centre of gravity and at right angles to the longitudinal axis have been determined. This allows deduction of the radius and moment of inertia about any axis through the centre of gravity and, consequently, about any axis in space.

As shown in the first series of experiments, the moments of inertia about four different axes through the centre of gravity and in a plane at right angles to the longitudinal axis of a body segment are about equal. This is true for the thigh and upper arm, for the leg and the arm and, therefore, also for the lower leg and forearm as a close approximation.

According to the general theory of the moments of inertia, if the moments of inertia about three axes in the same plane and through the same point O are equal, they are equal about all axes in this plane and through point O (pp. 57, 58). If the moment of inertia about the axis through point O and at right angles to this plane is the largest or the smallest of the moments of inertia, then all the moments of inertia about axes which form the same angle with a perpendicular to this plane are equal. $\varkappa'$ designates the radius of inertia about an axis in a plane through point O and $\varkappa''$ that about the perpendicular to this plane at O. The radius of inertia $\varkappa$ about any other axis through O and forming the angle γ with the perpendicular is:

$$\varkappa = \sqrt{\varkappa'^2 \sin^2 \gamma + \varkappa''^2 \cos^2 \gamma}.$$

This result is arrived at as follows. In Fig. 6, O is the origin of a system of co-ordinates fixed to the body, with the axes OX, OY, OZ.

OA is a straight line through the origin of the co-ordinates and forms the angles α, β, γ with the axes of co-ordinates.

x, y, z are the co-ordinates of a punctual mass m at P. PQ is at right angles to the line OA. The three points O, P and Q determine a right-angled triangle the hypotenuse of which is $OP = r$ and the sides of the right angle $PQ = \varrho$ and $OQ = p$. OQ is the projection of the segment OP on OA. This projection is equal to that of the broken line $OLPM$ on OA. The segments $OL = x$, $LM = y$ and $MP = z$ form with OA the angles α, β, γ. Therefore, the projection $OQ = p$ is the sum of the three projections $x \cos \alpha$, $y \cos \beta$ and $z \cos \gamma$

$$p = x \cos \alpha + y \cos \beta + z \cos \gamma$$

$OP = r$ can be expressed by its three co-ordinates:

$$r^2 = x^2 + y^2 + z^2.$$

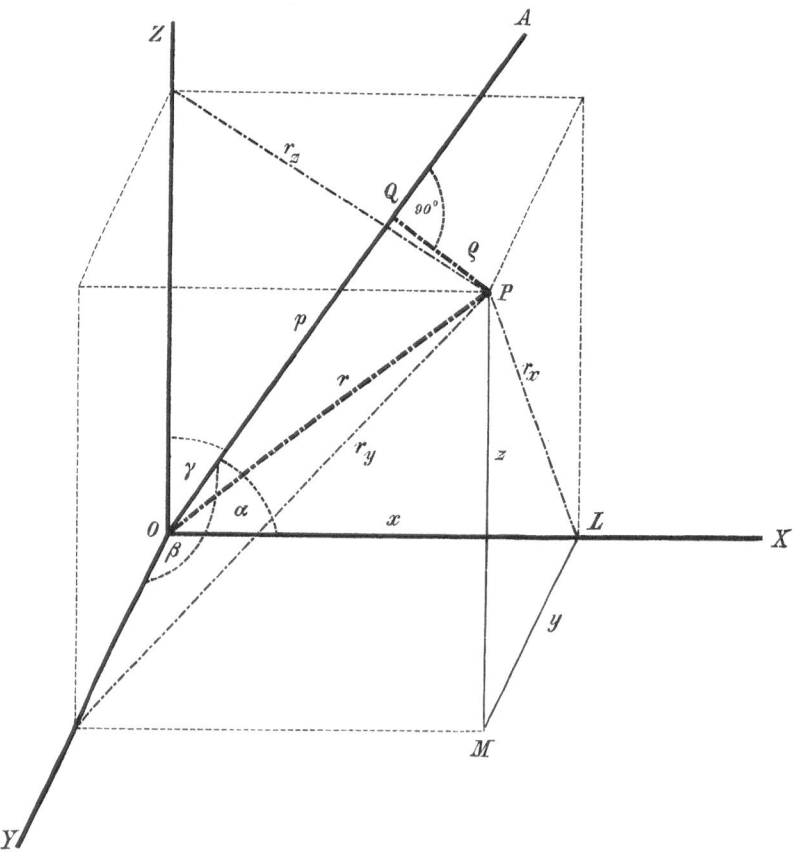

Fig. 6. Determination of the moment of inertia of a punctual mass P about an axis OA

Then, according to the Pythagorean rule:

$$\varrho^2 = (x^2 + y^2 + z^2) - (x \cos \alpha + y \cos \beta + z \cos \gamma)^2$$

or

$$\varrho^2 = x^2 (1 - \cos^2 \alpha) + y^2 (1 - \cos^2 \beta) + z^2 (1 - \cos^2 \gamma) \\ - 2 y z \cos \beta \cos \gamma - 2 z x \cos \gamma \cos \alpha - 2 x y \cos \alpha \cos \beta.$$

From the equation:

$$\cos^2 \alpha + \cos^2 \beta + \cos^2 \gamma = 1$$

it follows that:

$$1 - \cos^2 \alpha = \cos^2 \beta + \cos^2 \gamma \\ 1 - \cos^2 \beta = \cos^2 \gamma + \cos^2 \alpha \\ 1 - \cos^2 \gamma = \cos^2 \alpha + \cos^2 \beta.$$

Entering these values into the equation and arranging the members of the latter gives:

$$\varrho^2 = (y^2 + z^2) \cos^2 \alpha + (z^2 + x^2) \cos^2 \beta + (x^2 + y^2) \cos^2 \gamma \\ - 2 y z \cos \beta \cos \gamma - 2 z x \cos \gamma \cos \alpha - 2 x y \cos \alpha \cos \beta.$$

$y^2 + z^2$, $z^2 + x^2$ and $x^2 + y^2$ are the squares of the distances r_x, r_y and r_z between the point P and the three axes of co-ordinates. The mass m of point P is entered as a factor into the equation. Then:

$$m \varrho^2 = m r_x^2 \cdot \cos^2 \alpha + m r_y^2 \cdot \cos^2 \beta + m r_z^2 \cdot \cos^2 \gamma \\ - 2 m y z \cdot \cos \beta \cos \gamma - 2 m z x \cdot \cos \gamma \cos \alpha - 2 m x y \cdot \cos \alpha \cos \beta.$$

Since ϱ was the distance between point P and the line OA, $m \varrho^2$ is the moment of inertia of the punctual mass P about the axis OA. Moreover, $m r_x^2$, $m r_y^2$ and $m r_z^2$ are the moments of inertia of this punctual mass about the three axes of co-ordinates fixed to the body. The magnitudes $\cos \alpha$, $\cos \beta$ and $\cos \gamma$ are independent of the position of point P and maintain their value for any other punctual mass. If all the punctual masses of the body are added, the magnitudes $\cos^2 \alpha$, $\cos^2 \beta$, $\cos^2 \gamma$, $2 \cos \beta \cos \gamma$, $2 \cos \gamma \cos \alpha$ and $2 \cos \alpha \cos \beta$ can be considered as constant factors in the different sums. Then

$$\sum m\varrho^2 = \cos^2\alpha \sum m\,r_x^2 + \cos^2\beta \sum m\,r_y^2 + \cos^2\gamma \sum m\,r_z^2$$
$$- 2\cos\beta\cos\gamma \sum m\,y\,z - 2\cos\gamma\cos\alpha \sum m\,z\,x - 2\cos\alpha\cos\beta \sum m\,x\,y.$$

$\sum m\varrho^2$ is the moment of inertia T of the whole body about the axis OA and $\sum m\,r_x^2$, $\sum m\,r_y^2$ and $\sum m\,r_z^2$ are the moments of inertia of the whole body about the three axes of co-ordinates. Since the system of co-ordinates is assumed to be fixed to the body, the latter three moments of inertia are independent of the position of the axis OA and remain unchanged as long as the system of co-ordinates is not modified in the body. The moment of inertia about the axis OA depends on the direction of this axis and is a function of the three angles α, β, γ.

$\sum m\,y\,z$, $\sum m\,z\,x$ and $\sum m\,x\,y$ are independent of the position of the axis OA and maintain a constant value for any system of co-ordinates assumed to be fixed to the body. They are called the mass products of inertia of the body in relation to the three axes of co-ordinates.

If the three constant moments of inertia are designated as A, B, C and the three constant mass products of inertia as D, E, F, the equation of the moment of inertia about the axis OA becomes:

$$T = A\cos^2\alpha + B\cos^2\beta + C\cos^2\gamma - 2D\cos\beta\cos\gamma$$
$$- 2E\cos\gamma\cos\alpha - 2F\cos\alpha\cos\beta.$$

Thus, to determine the moment of inertia of a body about all the axes through a point O, it is necessary to know the three moments of inertia and the three mass products of inertia about the axes of a system of rectangular co-ordinates originating in O and fixed to the body in any arbitrary position.

Appropriate orientation of the system of co-ordinates simplifies the problem. For a certain position of this system, the three mass products of inertia are 0. Then, only the three moments of inertia about the axes of this particular system of co-ordinates must be known to determine any moment of inertia T.

This is clearly demonstrated by using a geometrical interpretation of the equation of T mentioned above. This interpretation was given by Cauchy and Poinsot was the first to recognize its importance in mechanics.

Division of the two members of the equation by the moment of inertia T gives:

$$1 = A\frac{\cos^2\alpha}{T} + B\frac{\cos^2\beta}{T} + C\frac{\cos^2\gamma}{T} - 2D\frac{\cos\beta\cos\gamma}{T}$$

$$- 2E\frac{\cos\gamma\cos\alpha}{T} - 2F\frac{\cos\alpha\cos\beta}{T}.$$

If from O a segment is taken over the axis OA with a length $\dfrac{1}{\sqrt{T}}$, the three co-ordinates of the extremity of this segment are:

$$x = \frac{1}{\sqrt{T}}\cos\alpha, \quad y = \frac{1}{\sqrt{T}}\cos\beta, \quad z = \frac{1}{\sqrt{T}}\cos\gamma,$$

OA forms with the axes of the co-ordinates the angles α, β, γ. Therefore:

$$\frac{\cos^2\alpha}{T} = x^2, \quad \frac{\cos^2\beta}{T} = y^2, \quad \frac{\cos^2\gamma}{T} = z^2,$$

$$\frac{\cos\beta\cos\gamma}{T} = yz, \quad \frac{\cos\gamma\cos\alpha}{T} = zx, \quad \frac{\cos\alpha\cos\beta}{T} = xy.$$

The equation above is changed into:

$$1 = Ax^2 + By^2 + Cz^2 - 2Dyz - 2Ezx - 2Fxy.$$

The relationship between the co-ordinates x, y, z of the extremity of the segment $\dfrac{1}{\sqrt{T}}$ on the axis OA is true whatever the direction of the axis OA. If x, y, z are variable co-ordinates of a point, this relationship represents the equation of a surface of the second order. This means that the extremities of all $\dfrac{1}{\sqrt{T}}$ long segments drawn from O on the corresponding axes lie over a surface of the second order. In no point of the surface can the three co-ordinates x, y, z become infinitely great. If it were so T should be 0. This is possible only if the whole body is reduced to a straight line or to a point. This eventuality is obviously unrealistic for our problem. Therefore, no point of the surface can be at infinity. That means that the surface of the second order must necessarily be an ellipsoid [8]. The ellipsoid is the only surface of the second order which is finite everywhere. The centre of the generally triaxial ellipsoid coincides with the origin of the co-ordinates.

---

[8] An ellipsoid is a closed surface all the cross sections of which are delineated by an ellipse which in some instances can become a circle. The surface of an egg, for instance, would be an ellipsoid if the longitudinal cross section of the egg was precisely an ellipse. It would then not be a general triaxial ellipsoid but rather an ellipsoid of revolution.

The following rule pertains: *If, on all the rays which originate from a fixed point O in a body, segments are taken starting from O and equal to the reciprocal values of the square root of the moment of inertia of the body about the corresponding ray considered as the axis, the extremities of these segments are on an ellipsoid. This ellipsoid is called the ellipsoid of inertia of the body about point O.* If point O is the centre of gravity of the body the ellipsoid is called central ellipsoid of inertia of the body.

This geometrical interpretation of the moments of inertia about the axes through a point illustrates the quantitative distribution of the moments of inertia of a body. Simultaneously it settles the whole theory of the distribution of the moments of inertia in a body by entering these moments of inertia into a well-known and worked-out geometrical theory, that of the surfaces of the second order. Any rule concerning the half axes of the ellipsoid is also valid for the moments of inertia. For example, if three half axes of the ellipsoid are at right angles to each other, the magnitude of one is a maximum, that of the second is a minimum and that of the third is an average. These three axes are called principal axes of the ellipsoid. Correspondingly if three straight lines through a point O are at right angles to each other, among the three moments of inertia about these lines, one has a maximum, the second a minimum and the third an average value. The three straight lines are called the principal axes of inertia of the point O. Relating the equation of the ellipsoid to the principal axes taken as axes of co-ordinates gives:

$$1 = A' x^2 + B' y^2 + C' z^2$$

in which A', B' and C' which are different from A, B and C have constant values in the new system of co-ordinates. Therefore, if the principal axes of the ellipsoid of inertia or principal axes of inertia for point O are taken as axes of co-ordinates the equation to determine T is simply:

$$T = A' \cos^2 \alpha + B' \cos^2 \beta + C' \cos^2 \gamma$$

in which A', B', C' are the moments of inertia about the three principal axes of inertia of point O. The three last members have dropped from the equation meaning that the three mass products of inertia about the principal axes of inertia are 0. The moments of inertia about the three principal axes of inertia are called principal moments of inertia and their radii principal radii of inertia of point O.

The three principal radii of inertia are $\varkappa_x$, $\varkappa_y$, $\varkappa_z$, the radius of inertia about the arbitrary axis OA is $\varkappa$ and the mass of the body is M. Then:

56

$$T = M\varkappa^2, \quad A' = M\varkappa_x^2, \quad B' = M\varkappa_y^2 \quad \text{und} \quad C' = M\varkappa_z^2.$$

Entering these values into the equation above and dividing by M gives:

$$\varkappa^2 = \varkappa_x^2 \cdot \cos^2\alpha + \varkappa_y^2 \cdot \cos^2\beta + \varkappa_z^2 \cdot \cos^2\gamma.$$

Determination of the moment and radius of inertia about any axis through the point O thus requires that three magnitudes be known: the three principal moments or three principal radii of inertia about point O.

If two of the three principal radii of inertia are equal, $\varkappa_y = \varkappa_x$, the equation becomes:

$$\varkappa^2 = \varkappa_x^2 (\cos^2\alpha + \cos^2\beta) + \varkappa_z^2 \cos^2\gamma$$

or, since $\cos^2\alpha + \cos^2\beta = 1 - \cos^2\gamma = \sin^2\gamma$,

$$\varkappa^2 = \varkappa_x^2 \cdot \sin^2\gamma + \varkappa_z^2 \cdot \cos^2\gamma.$$

In this instance, the ellipsoid of inertia is an ellipsoid of revolution. Its axis of rotation is the Z axis. All the half axes in the XY plane are equal. Then all radii and moments of inertia the axes of which are in the same plane as the two equal principal axes of inertia are also equal. One of the two unequal principal radii of inertia $\varkappa_x$ and $\varkappa_z$ is the greatest and the other the smallest of the radii of inertia in relation to axes through point O. In this particular case all the other radii of inertia can be calculated from these two principal radii of inertia.

As results from the preceding discussion, determination of the moments of inertia about all axes through a point O requires, above all, the search for the three principal axes of inertia. This is a geometrical problem which consists of determining the three principal axes of a given ellipsoid. Sometimes the result of this determination can be predicted. In many instances the shape and mass distribution of the body suggest that the moment of inertia about a well-determined straight line is a maximum or a minimum. For example, in a homogeneous body of revolution the axis of rotation is a principal axis of inertia for any point through which it passes.

It is often possible to predict that the moments of inertia about more than two axes through a point O and in one plane are equal. Then this is true about all axes through O and in the plane. (This appears immediately from the ellipsoid of inertia. Three equal half axes of the ellipsoid in one plane correspond to the three equal moments of inertia about three axes in one plane. The contours of the cross section of the ellipsoid in this plane are an ellipse and this ellipse has three equal half axes. This is possible only if the ellipse has become a circle and then all half axes in the plane considered are equal.) If it can also be predicted that the moment of inertia about the perpendicular to the plane at point O is a maximum or a minimum then the corresponding ellipsoid of inertia is an ellipsoid of revolution.

For the limbs of the human body and for their parts, the moments of inertia about four axes through the centre of gravity and in a plane at right angles to the long axis are about equal. At first glance, moreover, the shape of every body segment shows that the mass is at its most dense round the longitudinal axis. Consequently, the moment of inertia about the longitudinal axis of a body segment has about the smallest value. Here it is thus possible to predict that *the ellipsoid of inertia for the centre of gravity, i.e. the central ellipsoid of inertia, of every body segment is an ellipsoid of revolution. Therefore, determination of the moment of inertia about an axis at right angles to the longitudinal axis and of the moment of inertia about the longitudinal axis itself is sufficient to determine the moments of inertia about all axes through the centre of gravity.* $\varkappa_0'$ is the radius of inertia about an axis at right angles to the longitudinal axis and $\varkappa_0''$ that about the longitudinal axis itself. The radius of inertia $\varkappa_0$ about an axis through the centre of gravity and forming the angle γ with the longitudinal axis thus is, according to the equation on p. 57:

$$\varkappa_0 = \sqrt{\varkappa_0'^2 \sin^2 \gamma + \varkappa_0''^2 \cos^2 \gamma}.$$

Introducing the ellipsoid of inertia is important for the moments of inertia and their mechanical use. It illustrates the distribution of the moments of inertia about all axes through any point of a body. However, the absolute magnitude of a moment of inertia is somewhat difficult to see since the half axes of the ellipsoid give the reciprocal value of the square root of the radius of inertia. Consequently the proportions must be inverted. The greatest half axis of the ellipsoid corresponds to the smallest moment of inertia, the smallest of the three principal axes corresponds to the maximum and the greatest of the three principal axes to the minimum of the moment or radius of inertia.

More direct illustration of the magnitude of a moment of inertia is obtained by setting the length of the radius of inertia itself on every axis through O. The extremities of all these segments again form a surface which, however, presents the drawback of being none of the known surfaces of the second order.

The equation of this surface is (p. 57):

$$\varkappa^2 = \varkappa_x^2 \cos^2 \alpha + \varkappa_y^2 \cos^2 \beta + \varkappa_z^2 \cos^2 \gamma.$$

The two members can be multiplied by $\varkappa^2$. The co-ordinates x, y, z of this surface are such that:

$$\varkappa^2 = x^2 + y^2 + z^2$$

and

$$\varkappa^2 \cos^2 \alpha = x^2, \quad \varkappa^2 \cos^2 \beta = y^2, \quad \varkappa^2 \cos^2 \gamma = z^2.$$

Then the equation of the surface in rectangular co-ordinates is:

$$(x^2 + y^2 + z^2)^2 = \varkappa_x^2 x^2 + \varkappa_y^2 y^2 + \varkappa_z^2 z^2$$

in which $\varkappa_x$, $\varkappa_y$ and $\varkappa_z$ are the constant principal radii of inertia. Since here x, y, z appear at the fourth power, the surface is of the fourth order. This, however, is very close to an ellipsoid, that ellipsoid which is obtained if the three principal radii of inertia themselves (and not their reciprocal values) are used as principal axes. This ellipsoid is not at all similar to the ellipsoid of inertia. If a perpendicular is drawn from the centre of the ellipsoid to the plane tangent to the surface at every point of the ellipsoid, the extremities of these perpendiculars are generally outside the ellipsoid. They form a surface which envelops the ellipsoid and is called the surface of the extremities of the ellipsoid. This surface of the extremities has the equation above and is, therefore, identical with the surface formed by the extremities of the radii of inertia set on the axes. If the two principal axes of inertia $\varkappa_x$ and $\varkappa_y$ are equal, the ellipsoid, the principal axes of which are the principal radii of inertia, becomes an ellipsoid of revolution (like the ellipsoid of inertia) and its surface of the extremities similarily becomes an ellipsoid of revolution. The ellipsoid of revolution resulted from the revolution of the ellipse the principal axes of which were the two principal radii of inertia $\varkappa_x$ and $\varkappa_z$. Similarly the corresponding surface of the extremities results from the revolution of the curve of the extremities belonging to the ellipse. This is the curve linking the extremities of all the perpendiculars drawn from the centre of the ellipse to the tangents to the ellipse. In polar co-ordinates the equation of this curve is:

$$\varkappa^2 = \varkappa_x^2 \sin^2 \gamma + \varkappa_z^2 \cos^2 \gamma.$$

59

This is valid for the axes through the centre of gravity of all the segments of the human body. Thus, building this curve of the extremities for every case provides a complete insight into the magnitudes of the moments of inertia about all axes through the centre of gravity of a body segment.

The radius of inertia x_0' about an axis at right angles to the longitudinal axis and the radius of inertia x_0'' about the longitudinal axis are, in the present case, the two principal radii of inertia. Their magnitude has been taken as the average of their values on both sides of the body in Table 9. They are given in centimeters in Table 12.

The equations to calculate the radius of inertia x_0 about any axis through the centre of gravity and forming an acute angle γ with the longitudinal axis of the body segment thus are:

Thigh $\qquad x_0 = \sqrt{11.22^2 \cdot \sin^2 \gamma + 4.56^2 \cdot \cos^2 \gamma}$

Lower leg $\quad x_0 = \sqrt{9.41^2 \cdot \sin^2 \gamma + 3.09^2 \cdot \cos^2 \gamma}$

Arm $\qquad x_0 = \sqrt{7.87^2 \cdot \sin^2 \gamma + 2.77^2 \cdot \cos^2 \gamma}$

Forearm $\quad x_0 = \sqrt{10.84^2 \cdot \sin^2 \gamma + 2.73^2 \cdot \cos^2 \gamma}.$

The radii of inertia x_0 have been calculated for an angle γ changing by increments of $5°$ and are given in Table 13.

The data in Table 13 are valid for all axes which form the relevant acute angle γ with the longitudinal axis whatever plane they form with the latter.

To provide a clear picture of these radii of inertia, they are given in their natural size along the relevant axes in Figures 7–10. The curve which links the extremities of the segments indicates the radii of inertia about the intermediate axes. Figure 7 relates to the thigh, Figure 8 to the lower leg, Figure 9 to the upper arm and Figure 10 to the forearm + hand system. Imagining these diagrams rotated about the longitudinal axis of the body segment gives an overall view of the radii of inertia about all axes through the centre of gravity S of every body segment.

In all body segments, among all the moments of inertia about axes through the centre of gravity, that about the longitudinal axis is always the smallest. *The moment of inertia about the longitudinal axis of a segment of the human body is always the smallest which the body segment can have.* On the contrary, *the axes through the centre of gravity and at right angles to the longitudinal axis have the greatest moment of inertia.*

As far as the foot, head and trunk are concerned, the data obtained experimentally are not sufficiently reliable to deduce the moment of inertia about any axis through the centre of gravity. As long as sufficient data are not available, in these cases some likely assumptions may be useful.

Table 12. Principal radii of inertia (cm)

Body segments	$\varkappa_0'$	$\varkappa_0''$
Thigh	11.22	4.56
Lower leg	9.41	3.09
Arm	7.87	2.77
Forearm + hand	10.84	2.73

Table 13. Radii of inertia $\varkappa_0$ (cm) about axes through the centre of gravity and forming an angle γ with the longitudinal axis of the body segment (by increments of 5°)

Angle γ formed by the axis and the longitudinal axis of the body segment	Thigh	Lower leg	Upper arm	Forearm + hand
0°	4.56	3.09	2.77	2.73
5°	4.65	3.19	2.84	2.88
10°	4.89	3.45	3.05	3.28
15°	5.28	3.85	3.36	3.85
20°	5.75	4.34	3.74	4.51
25°	6.29	4.86	4.17	5.21
30°	6.86	5.41	4.61	5.91
35°	7.44	5.96	5.05	6.61
40°	8.01	6.50	5.49	7.28
45°	8.56	7.00	5.90	7.90
50°	9.08	7.48	6.29	8.49
55°	9.56	7.91	6.64	9.02
60°	9.98	8.29	6.95	9.49
65°	10.35	8.63	7.23	9.89
70°	10.66	8.91	7.46	10.23
75°	10.90	9.12	7.64	10.49
80°	11.08	9.28	7.77	10.69
85°	11.18	9.38	7.84	10.80
90°	11.22	9.41	7.87	10.84

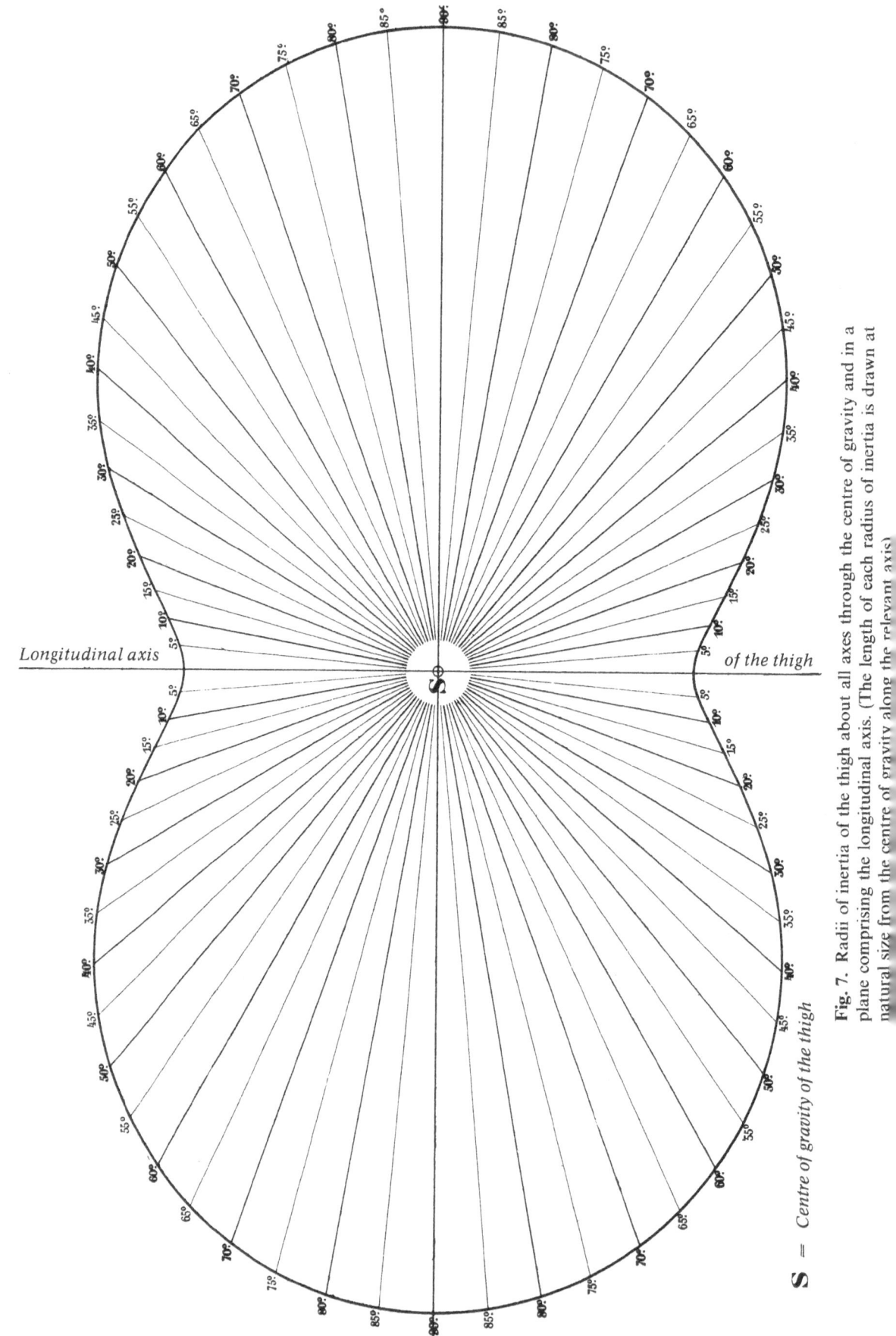

Longitudinal axis
of the thigh

S = Centre of gravity of the thigh

Fig. 7. Radii of inertia of the thigh about all axes through the centre of gravity and in a plane comprising the longitudinal axis. (The length of each radius of inertia is drawn at natural size from the centre of gravity along the relevant axis)

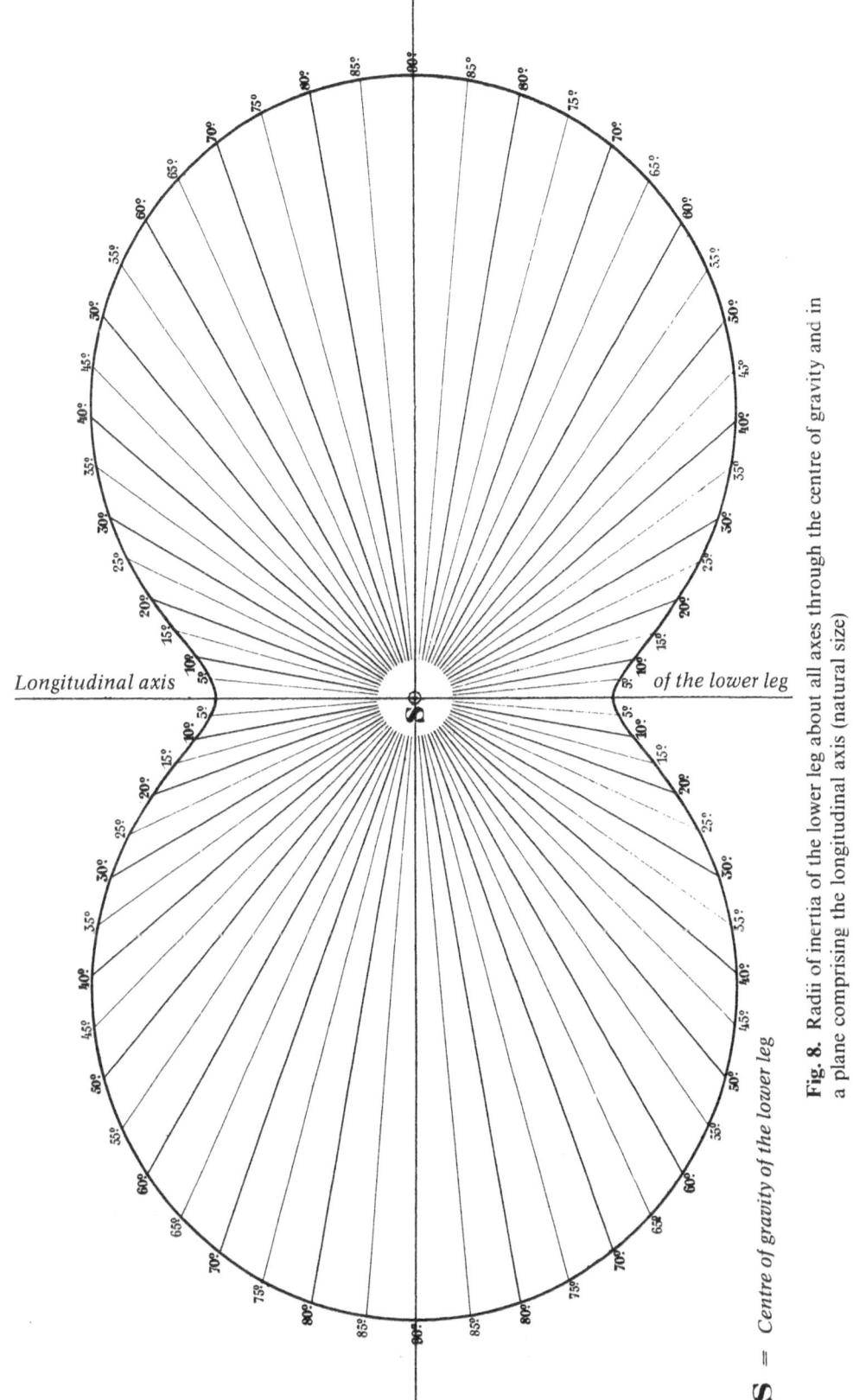

Longitudinal axis of the lower leg

Fig. 8. Radii of inertia of the lower leg about all axes through the centre of gravity and in a plane comprising the longitudinal axis (natural size)

S = *Centre of gravity of the lower leg*

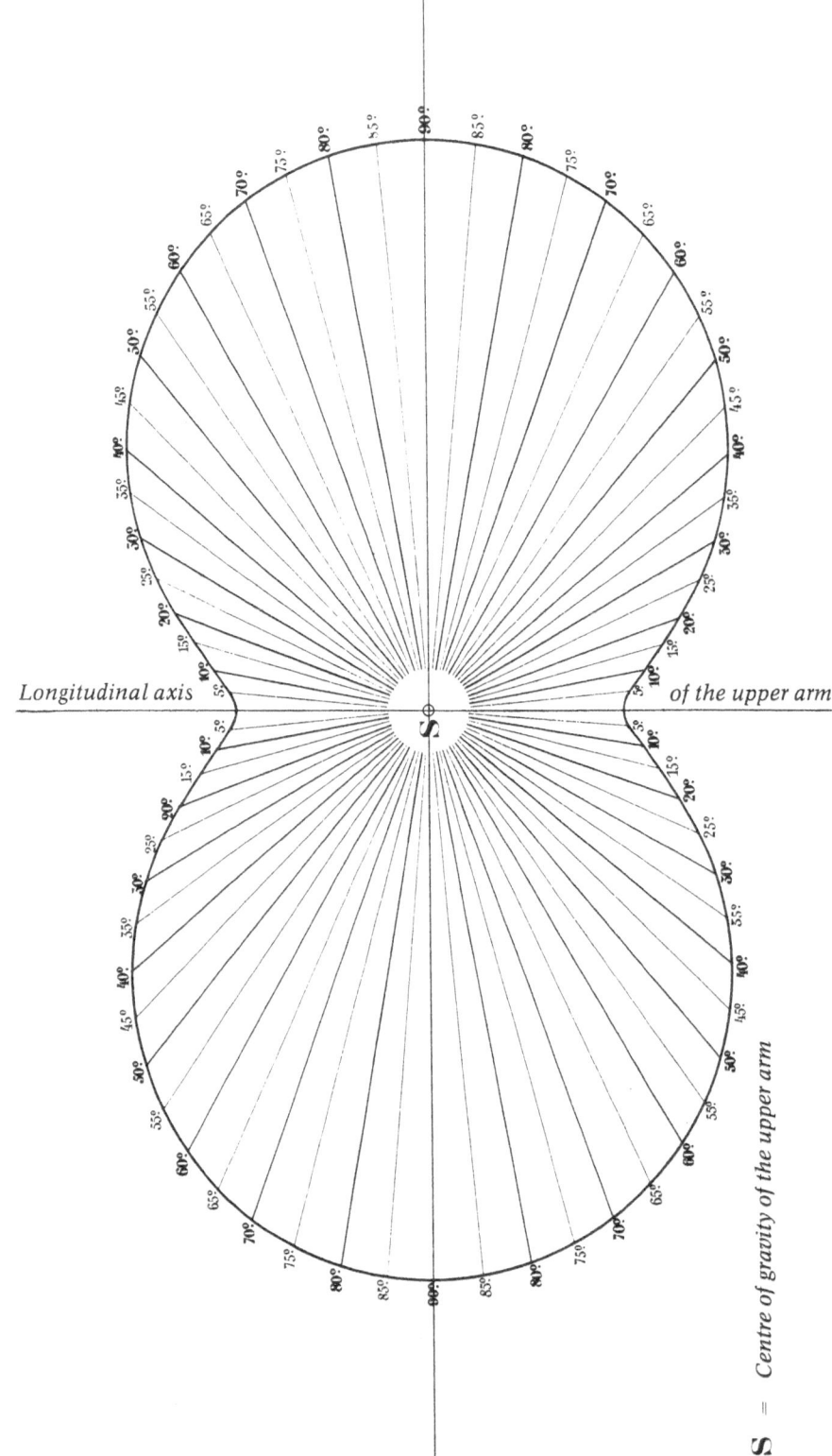

Longitudinal axis   of the upper arm

Fig. 9. Radii of inertia of the upper arm about all axes through the centre of gravity and in a plane comprising the longitudinal axis (natural size)

S = Centre of gravity of the upper arm

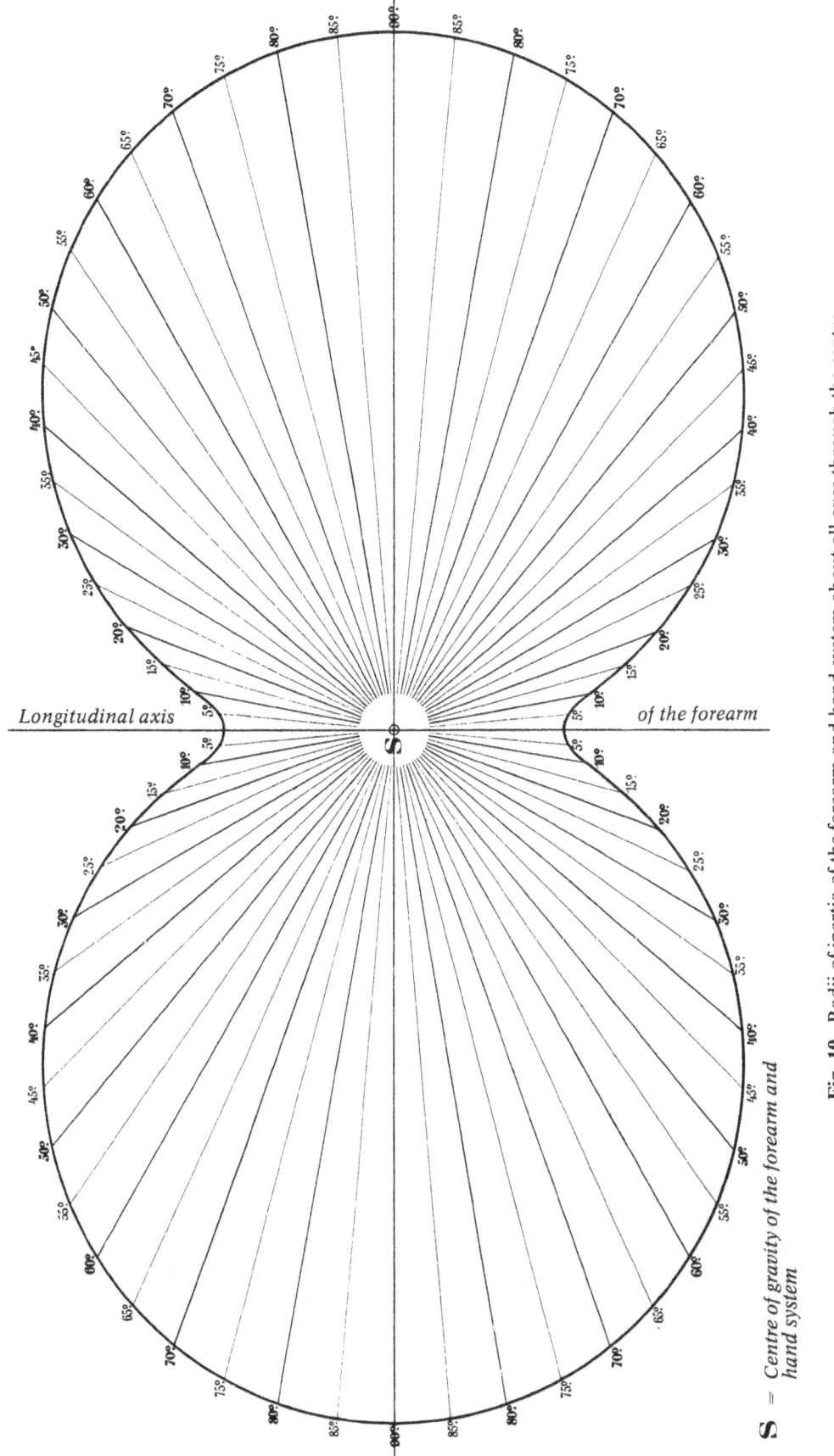

Fig. 10. Radii of inertia of the forearm and hand system about all axes through the centre of gravity of the system and in a plane comprising the longitudinal axis of the forearm (natural size)

S = *Centre of gravity of the forearm and hand system*

Longitudinal axis ———————— of the forearm

A rectangular system of co-ordinates can be fixed to the foot in such a way that, in the neutral position of the foot, the x-axis is at right angles to the longitudinal axis of the foot and also to the longitudinal axis of the lower leg and the y-axis is at right angles to the longitudinal axis of the foot but in the plane formed by the longitudinal axes of the foot and lower leg. Finally the z-axis coincides with the longitudinal axis of the foot, that is the line connecting the centre of the ankle and the tip of the foot. $\varkappa_x$, $\varkappa_y$ and $\varkappa_z$ are the radii of inertia about the three axes of co-ordinates. Only $\varkappa_x$ is given in Table 9. The average value of the right and left sides is $\varkappa_x = 5.94$ cm. The other radius of inertia of the foot was experimentally determined, not about the y-axis but about an axis which forms a 30° angle with the y-axis. Its average value is 6.23 cm. The shape of the foot suggests that the radius of inertia about the y-axis is even greater. $\varkappa_y$ thus is much greater than $\varkappa_x$. Consequently, the two radii of inertia of the foot about axes at right angles to the longitudinal axis are not equal. In this case the ellipsoid of inertia is presumably not an ellipsoid of revolution. Considering, for example, the radius of inertia of the lower leg about the axis at right angles to the longitudinal axis to be 9.41 cm and about an axis at 30° to the longitudinal axis to be 8.29 cm, it can be assumed that the radius of inertia of the foot about the y-axis is about 7 cm. If only the radii of inertia of the thigh about the axis at 30° to the longitudinal axis had been determined and found to be 9.98 cm, the same reasoning would give 11 cm as the radius of inertia about the axes at right angles to the longitudinal axis. This is close to the actual value: 11.22 cm. Presumably the value of 7 cm for the radius of inertia of the foot is a maximum. On the other hand, the radius of inertia $\varkappa_z$ about the z-axis, i.e. the longitudinal axis of the foot, can be considered as a minimum. Therefore, the three radii of inertia $\varkappa_x$, $\varkappa_y$, $\varkappa_z$ would be the three principal radii of inertia of the foot. By analogy with the lower leg, the radius of inertia $\varkappa_z$, for which there are even less clues than for $\varkappa_y$, can be evaluated at a third of the average value of the two other radii of inertia, that is 2 cm. To determine the radius of inertia $\varkappa$ about any axis through the centre of gravity of the foot and forming the angles α, β, γ with the three principal axes of inertia, the following equation pertains:

$$\varkappa^2 = 36 \cos^2 \alpha + 49 \cos^2 \beta + 4 \cos^2 \gamma$$

for which $\varkappa_x$ has been rounded up to 6 cm. The value of $\varkappa$ thus obtained is approximate. If this equation does not reflect exactly the actual conditions, it provides an approximate picture of the distribution of the moments of inertia of the foot until more precise determinations are available.

For the head we have even fewer data from direct measurement. We know only the radius of inertia about the coronal and horizontal axes through the centre of gravity when the head is maintained straight. The error is certainly small if provisionally the head is considered as a homogeneous sphere as far as its moments of inertia are concerned and all the radii of inertia about the axes through the centre of gravity are assumed to be equal.

It is different for the trunk. Here also we have determined the moment of inertia about one axis only, the axis through the centre of gravity and parallel to the hip axis. This is sufficient as far as rotation of the trunk about the hip axis is concerned but not to deal with the relative movement of the trunk in relation to the head. The trunk is the body segment mostly subjected to deformations and modifications in the internal distribution of its masses. Therefore, a general rule concerning its different moments of inertia can be enunciated only between certain limits. As long as the modifications of the moments of inertia resulting from changes in the shape of the trunk have not been analysed, it can be assumed, presumably without overstretching the risks of inaccuracy, that the same rule applies to the trunk as to the limbs as a result of its shape. The moments of inertia about all axes through the centre of gravity and at right angles to the longitudinal axis of the trunk thus would be equal. The moment of inertia about the longitudinal axis would be smaller than any other moment of inertia. The ellipsoid of inertia about the centre of gravity would be an ellipsoid of revolution the long axis of which coincides with the longitudinal axis of the trunk. In the trunk, however, the difference between the average diameter and the length is not so pronounced as in the limbs. Therefore, presumably the difference between the radius of inertia about the longitudinal axis and that about an axis through the centre of gravity and at right angles to the longitudinal axis is also smaller. The former may be about half the latter whereas for the limbs the ratio was one-third on average.

The radius of inertia $\varkappa_0'$ about the axis at right angles to the longitudinal axis is $\varkappa_0' = 16.73$ cm (Table 9). Therefore, the radius of inertia about the longitudinal axis would be $\varkappa_0'' = 8.5$ cm. For any other radius of inertia $\varkappa_0$ about an axis through the centre of gravity the following equation then would pertain:

$$\varkappa_0^2 = 280 \sin^2 \gamma + 72 \cos^2 \gamma,$$

in which γ is the angle formed by the relevant axis and the longitudinal axis of the trunk.

The assumptions made for the foot, head and trunk can hamper the validity of the results and should be confirmed by further research. However, the results derived from these assumptions, together with those empirically obtained for the limbs and which are thus more reliable, provide an orientating overall view of the quantitative distribution of the moments of inertia in all the important segments of the human body. From this point of view even the results obtained for the foot, head and trunk are of some value as long as nothing more reliable is available.

Deduction of the Moments of Inertia
About Any Axis in Space

𝔄 fter the moments of inertia about all axes through the centre of gravity of every body segment have been determined, that about any axis in space outside the centre of gravity can also be found. To this end it must be repeated (p. 12) that the moment of inertia T about any axis in space at a distance e from the centre of gravity of the body can be expressed by the moment of inertia T_0 about the axis parallel to the first according to the equation:

$$T = T_0 + M e^2$$

in which M is the mass of the body. $\varkappa$ designates the radius of inertia for T whereas $\varkappa_0$ designates the radius of inertia for T_0. The following relationship exists between these two radii of inertia and the distance e between the axis and the centre of gravity:

$$\varkappa^2 = \varkappa_0^2 + e^2.$$

The moment and radius of inertia about any axis outside the centre of gravity thus are always greater than those about the axis parallel to the first and through the centre of gravity.

To analyse the movement of the different segments of the human body in relation to each other, the moments of inertia about joint axes are mainly considered. Since the centre of gravity of every body segment lies on its longitudinal axis, the moment of inertia about the longitudinal axis does not change when going from the centre of gravity to the centre of one of the adjacent joints. However, all the other moments of inertia become greater. But again all the moments of inertia about such joint axes which are at right angles to the longitudinal axis of the body segment are equal. All these axes are at the same distance from the centre of gravity, that is the distance between the centre of gravity and the centre of the joint. $\varkappa'$ is the radius of inertia about a joint axis at right angles to the longitudinal axis, $\varkappa''$ is the radius of inertia about the longitudinal axis whereas $\varkappa_0'$ and $\varkappa_0''$ are the radii of inertia about two axes through the centre of gravity, one parallel to the joint axis and the other to the longitudinal axis. Therefore:

$$\varkappa'^2 = \varkappa_0'^2 + e^2 \quad \text{and} \quad \varkappa''^2 = \varkappa_0''^2$$

(Actually the axes for $\varkappa''$ and $\varkappa_0''$ are identical, i.e. the longitudinal axis).

The radius of inertia about any axis through a point can be deduced from the three or two principal radii of inertia of this point. This rule is valid for any point and not only for the centre of gravity. Therefore, the radius of inertia $\varkappa$ about any axis which forms an angle γ with the longitudinal axis of the body segment can be obtained in the same way, from the two principal radii of inertia. $\varkappa'$ and $\varkappa''$ are these principal radii of inertia about the centre of the joint as $\varkappa_0'$ and $\varkappa_0''$ are the principal radii of inertia about the centre of gravity. Thus:

$$\varkappa^2 = \varkappa'^2 \cdot \sin^2 \gamma + \varkappa''^2 \cdot \cos^2 \gamma.$$

If the principal radii of inertia of the centre of gravity are used:

$$\varkappa^2 = (\varkappa_0'^2 + e^2) \sin^2 \gamma + \varkappa_0''^2 \cos^2 \gamma.$$

Since $\varkappa_0'^2 \sin^2 \gamma + \varkappa_0''^2 \cos^2 \gamma = \varkappa_0^2$ in which $\varkappa_0$ is the radius of inertia $\varkappa$ about the parallel axis through the centre of gravity, the equation can be written as follows:

$$\varkappa^2 = \varkappa_0^2 + e^2 \sin^2 \gamma.$$

This equation can be used advantageously if the radii of inertia about all axes through the centre of gravity have been calculated previously.

To give an example of the change in the moments of inertia when moving to the centre of a joint, we have calculated the radii of inertia of the upper arm about the centre of the humeral head. The average distance between the centre of the humeral head and the centre of gravity of the upper arm is 11.84 cm (Table 9). Therefore, the following equation enables the radii of inertia $\varkappa$ about the centre of the humeral head to be calculated:

$$\varkappa = \sqrt{(7.87^2 + 11.84^2) \sin^2 \gamma + 2.77^2 \cos^2 \gamma}.$$

If the previously calculated value of the radii of inertia $\varkappa_0$ of the centre of gravity is used (Table 13):

$$\varkappa = \sqrt{\varkappa_0^2 + 11.84^2 \cdot \sin^2 \gamma}.$$

Table 14. Radii of inertia $\varkappa$ (cm) of the upper arm about axes through the centre of the humeral head and forming an angle γ with the longitudinal axis (increments by 5°)

γ	$\varkappa$	γ	$\varkappa$	γ	$\varkappa$
0°	2.77	35°	8.45	65°	12.94
5°	3.02	40°	9.38	70°	13.39
10°	3.68	45°	10.24	75°	13.75
15°	4.55	50°	11.04	80°	14.01
20°	5.51	55°	11.75	85°	14.17
25°	6.51	60°	12.39	90°	14.22
30°	7.50				

The values of $\varkappa$ thus obtained are given in Table 14.

The radii of inertia are reproduced at natural size along the corresponding axes in Figure 11. Simultaneously the radii of inertia of the centre of gravity are indicated as delineated by a dotted curve. Comparison of the two curves shows that the moments of inertia about the axes at right angles to the longitudinal axis of the body segment become significantly greater when moving to the centre of the joint whereas the moment of inertia in relation to the longitudinal axis remains unchanged. A much bigger difference appears between the moment of inertia about the longitudinal axis and the moments of inertia about joint axes at right angles to the longitudinal axis of the upper arm. The same ratio between the moments of inertia is found in every body segment. *This difference explains why the muscles which rotate a body segment about its longitudinal axis are much less bulky than the flexor and extensor muscles. For the same reason and because of their oblique insertion, their torque about the longitudinal axis which is the axis of rotation is small.* As a result of the smaller moment of inertia every body segment offers a significantly smaller resistance to rotation about its longitudinal axis than to movement about an axis at right angles to the longitudinal axis.

For the foot, we obtained three different principal radii of inertia of the centre of gravity. Therefore, three different principal radii of inertia should be obtained for every other point of the body segment. Particularly the three principal radii of inertia $\varkappa'$, $\varkappa''$, $\varkappa'''$ of the centre of the ankle joint are:

$$\varkappa'^2 = \varkappa_0'^2 + e^2, \quad \varkappa''^2 = \varkappa_0''^2 + e^2 \quad \text{and} \quad \varkappa'''^2 = \varkappa_0'''^2$$

if $\varkappa_0'$, $\varkappa_0''$ and $\varkappa_0'''$ are the three principal radii of inertia (the last in relation to the longitudinal axis) of the centre of gravity and e the

71

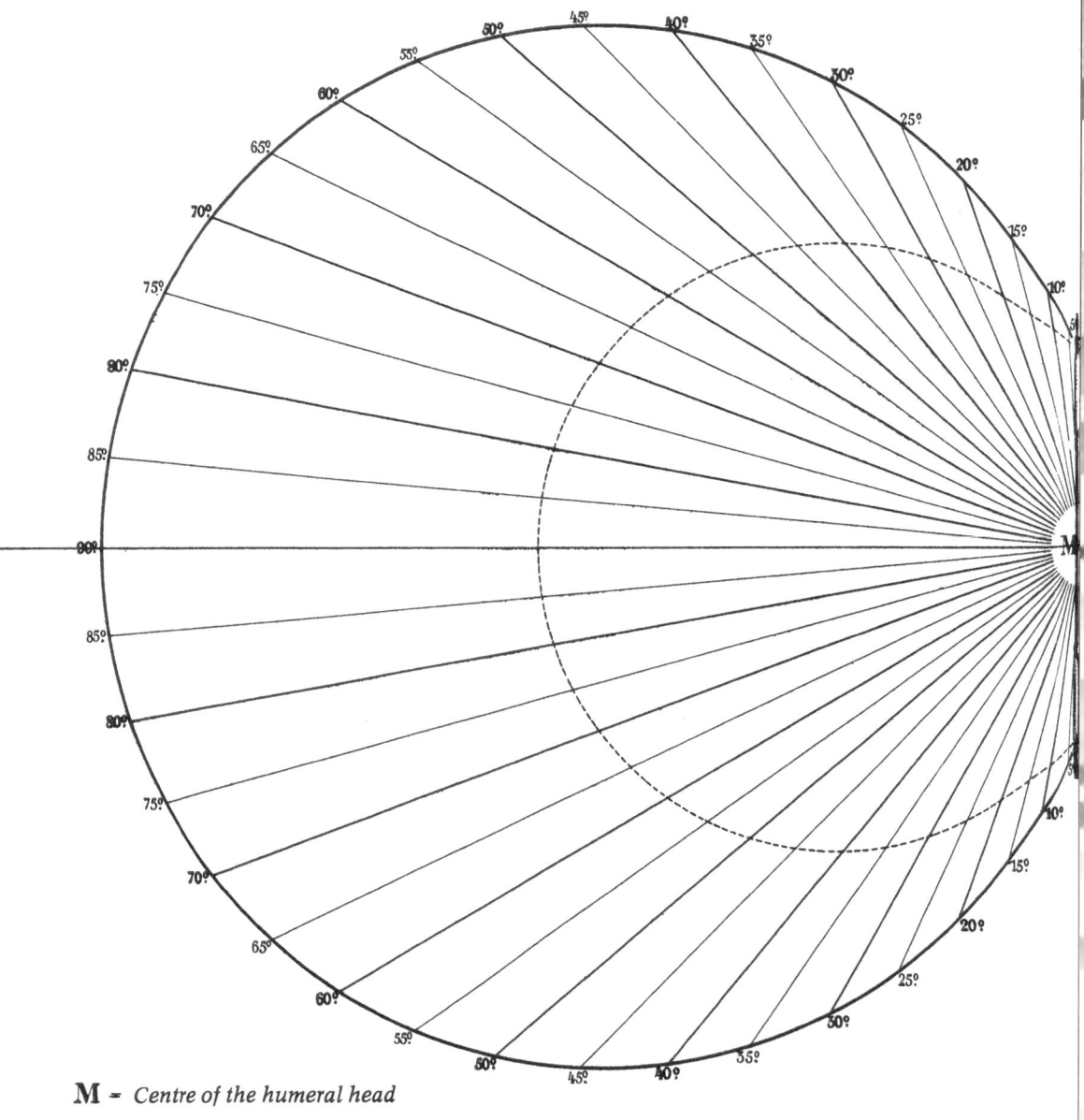

M = *Centre of the humeral head*

Fig. 11. Radii of inertia of the upper arm about all axes through the centre of the humeral head and in a plane comprising the longitudinal axis. To allow for comparison, the radii of inertia of the upper arm about all axes through the centre of gravity are given. They are delineated by the dotted curve (natural size)

72

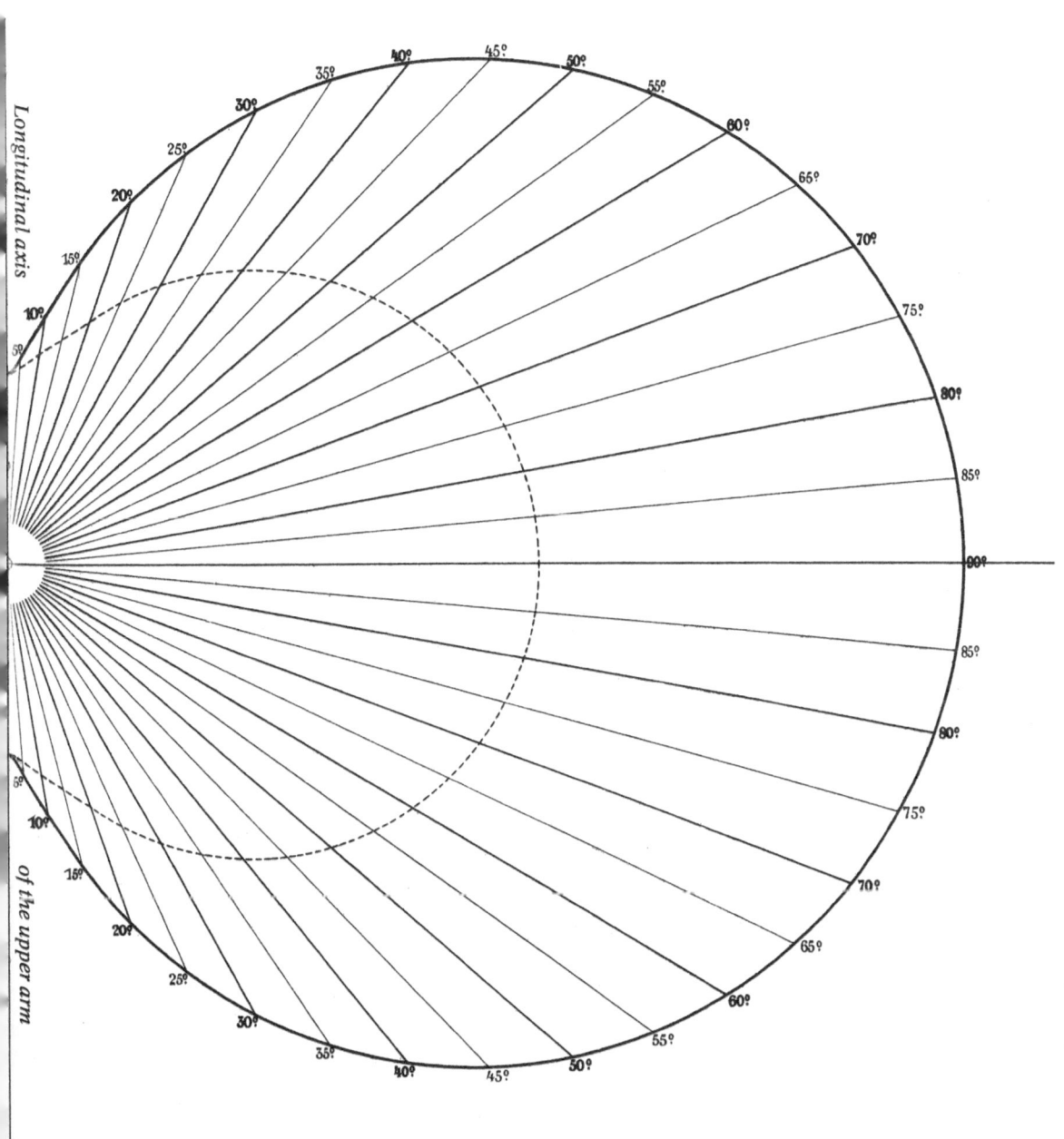

distance between the centre of gravity of the foot and the centre of the ankle joint. Then for any radius of inertia $\varkappa$ about an axis through the centre of the ankle joint and forming the angles α, β, γ with the three principal radii of inertia, the following equation pertains:

$$\varkappa^2 = (\varkappa_0'^2 + e^2)\cos^2\alpha + (\varkappa_0''^2 + e^2)\cos^2\beta + \varkappa_0'''^2\cos^2\gamma.$$

It often occurs that the moments of inertia of a body segment about axes belonging to joints which have no direct connection with the body segment are needed. To analyse the oscillations of the lower leg + foot system about the knee, for example, the moment of inertia of the foot in any position to the lower leg about the axis of the knee is needed. In such instances either it must be found how far the centre of gravity of each body segment is from the axis of rotation as a result of the reciprocal position of the body segments, or the moment of inertia of the system of body segments about the axis through the total centre of gravity of the system and parallel to the relevant joint axis can be sought (see page 44) and the distance between this joint axis and the centre of gravity determined. The first manner is simpler.

Example of Application of the Moments of Inertia Thus Found: Determination of the Period of Oscillation of the Leg at Different Degrees of Flexion

$\mathfrak{A}$n example will show how the results thus obtained are used; we chose to determine the period of oscillation of the leg with the knee at different degrees of flexion.

In Figure 12, as in Figure 3:

H is the centre of the hip joint,
K that of the knee joint,
S_1 the centre of gravity of the thigh,
S_2 that of the lower leg + foot system,
s_1 the length of the segment KS_1,
s_2 that of the segment KS_2,
$\varkappa_1$ the radius of inertia of the thigh,
$\varkappa_2$ that of the lower leg + foot system,
 each of them about an axis through
 the centre of gravity S_1 or S_2
 and parallel to the axis of the knee,
m_1 the mass of the thigh,
m_2 that of the lower leg + foot system,
t the length of the thigh and
ω the angle of flexion of the knee.

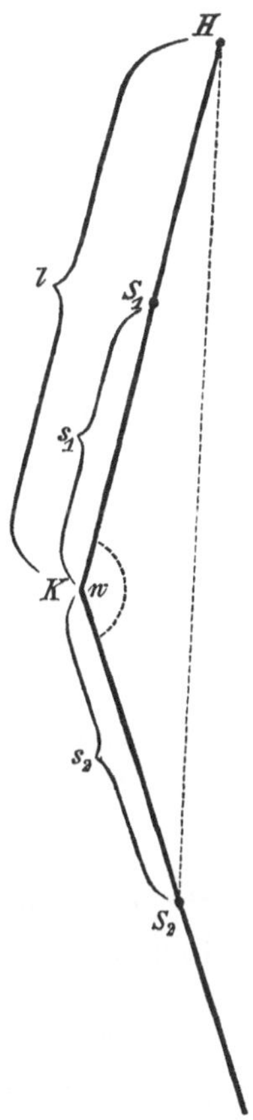

Fig. 12. Determination of the period of oscillation of the leg with the knee flexed

The centre of gravity S_1 is at a distance $l - s_1$ from the centre of the hip joint H and the centre of gravity S_2 at a distance from H equal to

$$\sqrt{l^2 + s_2^2 - 2\,l\,s_2\cos\omega}\,.$$

Consequently, if the axis of the knee joint is fixed and at right angles to the plane determined by the three points S_1, K, S_2 then the moment of inertia of the thigh about an axis through the centre of the hip H and parallel to the axis of the knee, is

$$m_1\left[\varkappa_1^2 + (l - s_1)^2\right]$$

and the moment of inertia of the lower leg + foot system about the same axis is

$$m_2\left[\varkappa_2^2 + (l^2 + s_2^2 - 2\,l\,s_2\cos\omega)\right].$$

The moment of inertia of the leg about this coronal axis through the centre of the hip is

$$m_1\left[\varkappa_1^2 + (l - s_1)^2\right] + m_2\left[\varkappa_2^2 + (l^2 + s_2^2 - 2\,l\,s_2\cos\omega)\right]$$

or

$$m_1\,\varkappa_1^2 + m_2\,\varkappa_2^2 + m_1\,(l - s_1)^2 + m_2\,(l^2 + s_2^2 - 2\,l\,s_2\cos\omega),$$

in which $m_1\,\varkappa_1^2$ and $m_2\,\varkappa_2^2$ are the moments of inertia of the thigh and of the lower leg + foot system about axes through the centres of gravity and parallel to the axis through the hip. These moments of inertia were determined previously.

Consequently, according to the well-known rule of the pendulum (p. 28), the period of oscillation τ of the leg suspended from a coronal axis through the hip joint, for small amplitudes, is:

$$\tau = \pi\sqrt{\frac{m_1\,\varkappa_1^2 + m_2\,\varkappa_2^2 + m_1\,(l - s_1)^2 + m_2\,(l^2 + s_2^2 - 2\,l\,s_2\cos\omega)}{g\left[m_1\,(l - s_1) + m_2\,\sqrt{l^2 + s_2^2 - 2\,l\,s_2\cos\omega}\right]}}\,.$$

If the data in Table 9 (p. 42) for the left leg are used, the following values must be entered into the equation:

$$m_1 = 4\,810, \quad \varkappa_1 = 11.43, \quad s_1 = 20.75, \quad l = 36.65,$$
$$m_2 = 2\,800, \quad \varkappa_2 = 15.10, \quad s_2 = 21.94, \quad g = 981.11 \text{ (for Leipzig)}.$$

76

Table 15. Periods of oscillation of the left leg with the knee at different degrees of flexion (for small amplitudes)

Angle of flexion ω	Period of oscillation τ (s)	ω	τ	ω	τ
180° (extension)	0.711	150°	0.701	115°	0.664
		145°	0.697	110°	0.657
175°	0.711	140°	0.693	105°	0.6495
170°	0.710	135°	0.688	100°	0.641
165°	0.709	130°	0.683	95°	0.633
160°	0.7065	125°	0.677	90° (flexion at right angles)	0.624
155°	0.704	120°	0.671		

The periods of oscillation τ of the leg have thus been calculated with the knee flexing from full extension ($\omega = 180°$) to the right angle ($\omega = 90°$) by increments of 5°. They are given in Table 15.

The period of oscillation is the shorter, the more the knee is flexed. The diminution of the period of oscillation with the decrease of the angle of flexion, however, is very slow. As a whole, between extension and flexion at 90° the diminution of the period of oscillation is less than 0.1 s. These periods are valid only for small amplitudes. When the amplitudes are larger, as for example during gait, the periods of oscillation must be corrected. α designates the half-amplitude (or angular range) of the pendulum, that is the angle formed by the plane through the axis of oscillation and the centre of gravity, and the vertical plane through the axis of oscillation when the centre of gravity is at its furthest from the vertical plane. The precise period of oscillation τ' is expressed as follows, using the value τ valid for small amplitudes only:

$$\tau' = \tau \left[1 + \left(\frac{1}{2}\right)^2 \sin^2\frac{\alpha}{2} + \left(\frac{1\cdot 3}{2\cdot 4}\right)^2 \sin^4\frac{\alpha}{2} + \left(\frac{1\cdot 3\cdot 5}{2\cdot 4\cdot 6}\right)^2 \sin^6\frac{\alpha}{2} + \cdots \right].$$

The precision with which the value of τ can be determined decides up to which member of the equation in the brackets the calculation must be carried out.

Summary

The introduction gives a definition of the moment of inertia and explains its importance for the dynamics of the human body. It is not sufficient to know the mass and position of the centre of gravity of a body segment to be able to predict the behaviour of the latter towards forces which tend to rotate it about an axis. After the mass and the position of the centre of gravity of a body have been determined, determination of its moment of inertia about any axis in space makes the body a known object of the movement. Two bodies which have the same mass, position of their centre of gravity and moments of inertia are equivalent in a dynamic sense whatever the difference of their shape and constitution may be. Finding the moments of inertia of the human body and of its segments thus is as necessary as determining the action of the different muscles.

The moments of inertia of the segments of the human body cannot be found by calculation alone. They must be deduced empirically. At first we measured the period of oscillation of a body segment suspended from an axis through a joint, its mass and the distance between its centre of gravity and the axis of oscillation. These three data were sufficient to determine the moment of inertia about a straight line through the centre of gravity and parallel to the axis of oscillation. However, direct external measurement of the distance between the axis and the centre of gravity is not sufficiently accurate to determine the moment of inertia. Therefore, in a second series of experiments, we modified the method and measured the periods of oscillation in relation to two parallel axes which determined a plane comprising the centre of gravity. These two periods of oscillation together with the distance between the two axes and the mass of the body segment are sufficient to determine the moment of inertia about the axis through the centre of gravity and parallel to the axes of oscillation. They also enable the distances between the centre of gravity and the two parallel axes of oscillation to be determined precisely.

We determined the moments of inertia of every important body segment generally about two axes through its centre of gravity, one at right angles to the longitudinal axis of the body segment and the other coinciding with the longitudinal axis itself. It was sufficient to determine one axis at right angles to the longitudinal axis since it appeared that, as a rule, the moments of inertia about all axes through the centre of gravity and at right angles to the longitudinal axis are about equal.

The following conclusions could be drawn:

1. For all segments of the human body the ratio of the radius of inertia about any axis through the centre of gravity and at right angles to the longitudinal axis, to the length of the body segment is the same. Its constant value is about 0.30.
2. For the thigh, lower leg and upper arm (and presumably also for the forearm), the ratio of the radius of inertia about the longitudinal axis, to the average diameter of the body segment is the same. Its constant value is about 0.35.

These two rules enable the moment of inertia to be determined even in vivo. μ designates the almost constant ratio of the mass of a body segment to the total mass M, l the length of this body segment and d its average diameter. Then its moment of inertia T_0' about any axis through its centre of gravity and at right angles to its longitudinal axis is

$$T_0' = 0{,}30^2 \, \mu \, M \, l^2$$

and the moment of inertia about the longitudinal axis is

$$T_0'' = 0{,}35^2 \, \mu \, M \, d^2$$

in which the total mass M of the human body and the magnitudes l and d can be measured directly in vivo.

From these two moments of inertia, every other moment of inertia about any axis can be calculated (except for the foot). If this axis forms an angle γ with the longitudinal axis, the corresponding axis of inertia T_0 is

$$T_0 = T_0' \sin^2 \gamma + T_0'' \cos^2 \gamma.$$

To determine all moments of inertia of the foot about the axes through its centre of gravity, three moments of inertia are necessary, one T_0' about the axis at right angles to the plane formed by the longitudinal axes of the foot and lower leg, when the foot is in the neutral position, the second T_0'' about the axis which is in this plane and at right angles to the longitudinal axis of the foot and the third T_0''' about the longitudinal axis of the foot itself. If α, β, γ are the angles formed by another axis through the centre of gravity and the three axes corresponding to these three moments of inertia, the moment of inertia T_0 about this axis is:

$$T_0 = T_0' \cos^2 \alpha + T_0'' \cos^2 \beta + T_0''' \cos^2 \gamma.$$

For the thigh, lower leg, upper arm and forearm + hand system, the moments of inertia have been calculated about all the axes through the centre of gravity inclined to each other by 5° and the lengths of the corresponding radii of inertia have been drawn in Figures 7–10. These figures show that the moment of inertia about the longitudinal axis of one of the body segments is the smallest among all the moments of inertia about axes through the centre of gravity.

The moments of inertia about all other axes in space can be deduced from the moments of inertia about axes through the centre of gravity. If e is the distance between an axis A and the centre of gravity and T_0 the moment of inertia of the body about an axis through the centre of gravity and parallel to the first, the moment of inertia T about the axis A is:

$$T = T_0 + m e^2$$

in which m is the mass of the body segment. As an example, the moments of inertia of the upper arm about all the axes through the shoulder joint forming with each other angles of 5° were calculated and the corresponding radii of inertia drawn in Figure 11. The moment of inertia about the longitudinal axis remains unchanged when moving from the centre of gravity to the centre of the joint whereas all other moments of inertia about axes similarly orientated become greater. The moment of inertia about the longitudinal axis is thus the smallest possible of this body segment. This explains that the flexor and extensor muscles which simultaneously exert a rotatory effect about the longitudinal axis of a body segment have such a small component of rotation and exert such a small torque about the longitudinal axis. Moreover, the muscles which evoke only rotation about the longitudinal axis are relatively small.

Finally the period of oscillation of the leg with the knee at different degrees of flexion is calculated as an example of the utilization of the moments of inertia thus found.

Index

W. Braune, O. Fischer

The Human Gait

Translated from the German by P. Maquet,
R. Furlong

1987. 101 figures, 120 tables. X, 440 pages.
ISBN 3-540-15270-9

Contents: Experiments on Man, Loaded and
Unloaded. – The Movement of the Total Centre
of Gravity and the External Forces. – Considera-
tions on the Final Aims of Research and
General Survey of the Movements of the Lower
Extremities. – On the Movement of the Foot
and the Forces Acting on it. – Kinematics of the
Swing of the Leg. – On the Influence of Gravity
and the Muscles of the Swinging Movement of
the Leg. – Subject Index.

Braune and Fischer's classic analysis of the
human gait has never been equalled in its
comprehensiveness and accuracy. The authors
entered in a rectangular system of co-ordinates
the centers of gravity of the body and of the
different segments of the body, together with the
centers of the different joints of their experimen-
tal subjects, for the successive phases of gait.
They calculated the external and internal forces
involved in walking and described the kinematics and kinetics of the movement in detail. This
work, although often cited, is almost unknown
in the English-speaking countries and is difficult
to find even in the original German. It will be of
tremendous help to all those in the fields of
anatomy, physiology, orthopedic surgery, rheu-
matology and rehabilitation medicine, who are
interested in normal and abnormal walking.

Springer-Verlag
Berlin Heidelberg New York
London Paris Tokyo

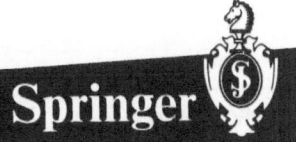

Springer

W. Braune, O. Fischer

On the Centre of Gravity of the Human Body

as Related to the Equipment of the German Infantry Soldier

Translated from the German by P. Maquet, R. Furlong

1985. 33 figures, 51 tables. VII, 96 pages. ISBN 3-540-13216-3

From the reviews:
"...should appeal to those engaged in the study of body statics and mechanics. It is an authentic and deeply authoritative work whose data remain the most precise on the subject to date. It illustrates how ingenuity, energy, and exactitude can solve problems in biophysical science. We look forward to *The Human Gait,* by the same authors (and translators)..." *Journal of the American Medical Association*

J. Wolff

The Law of Bone Remodelling

Translated from the German by P. Maquet, R. Furlong

1986. 95 figures. XII, 126 pages. ISBN 3-540-16281-X

Contents: Concept of the Law of Bone Remodelling. – The Internal Architecture of Normal Bone and Its Mathematical Significance. – Remodelling of the Internal Architecture and External Shape of Bones. – Functional Shape of Bone. – On the Remodelling Force and Its Therapeutic Use. – Consequences Drawn from the Law of Bone Remodelling. – Appendices. – References.

Springer-Verlag
Berlin Heidelberg New York
London Paris Tokyo

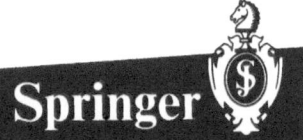